ONE HUNDRED PRAYERS

By
Anthony Eckshar MD

Readers are welcome to comment to the author at

anthonyeckshar@gmail.com.

TABLE OF CONTENTS

DEDICATION

Ad Majorem Dei Gloriam – *For the greater glory of God.*

To my wife Jean, the closest thing to an angel on Earth, my partner *outside* the ICU, that keeps me healthy, happy and on the right path.

To the best ICU team I could hope to be part of, most of all, the ever-tolerant and kindhearted nurses.

To the long-suffering patients and their families whom we served to the best of our abilities.

INTRODUCTION

On March 20, 2020, anticipating the struggle of a lifetime against Covid pneumonia in the intensive care unit (ICU) where I worked, I promised to say a prayer a day for a hundred days. I imagine now that God may have smiled at my naïve optimism. Eventually, I recorded over 270 prayers and my praying days continued long after the worse of Covid were far behind. The *context* of my prayers will be alien to those who don't work in the ICU, so I thought I should first introduce some medical terminology and describe *why* I decided to pray as the pandemic approached. Once that's done, I'll share the prayers and stories surrounding them.

I am a Critical Care physician, sixty years old when this story began, happily married for 35 years with two grown-up kids. I'm a Christian, but not a very good one by some criteria. For one thing, I'm not church-going – tough to get into that routine when you work three out of-four Sundays. I didn't regularly read the Bible. I had doubts about how strong my faith was. *Would it hold up under adversity?* I was about to find out.

My six partners and I staff the medical ICU at a large hospital in metropolitan Phoenix, Arizona. Our ICU is comprised of a 50-bed hospital ward and a healthcare team specialized in taking care of patients with life-threatening medical illnesses like severe pneumonia, heart attack and stroke. ICU patients often require life support unavailable in any other unit of the hospital, implemented by mechanical ventilators, dialysis machines, heart support pumps and monitor probes placed directly into the brain. The ICU team takes care of the sickest patients around the clock and also has the duty of "running codes" (providing advanced cardiac life support (ACLS) to patients who lose their pulse or stop breathing). So you can understand why one of my partners or I have to be physically present in our ICU 24 hours per day, 365 days per year.

Our ICU team was built on mutual respect and friendship. Based on past experience, I knew we could handle almost any emergency together. My partners (Joyce, Mayfield and the others), the nurses, respiratory therapists who run our ventilators, IV access team, social workers, echocardiography techs, housekeepers – *everyone without whom an ICU doctor really can't get anything done* – were smart, cheerful, compassionate and hard-working with few exceptions. We had good camaraderie and high morale, which we would soon need more than ever, as we were destined to bear witness to the deaths of over four hundred people from Covid pneumonia despite our best efforts to save them.

COVID-19 is caused by a type of virus called a coronavirus because projections on its surface that allow it to infect cells in the human throat and lungs surround the virus in the shape of a "corona" or crown. Covid spread from bats to humans in the winter of 2019, but that wasn't the first time a bat coronavirus caused a lethal outbreak in humans. I'm going to briefly digress to tell the story of SARS because it weighed heavy on my mind in March 2020.

In November 2002, a mysterious cluster of highly-contagious pneumonia cases broke out in Guangdong Province, China – a disease that would eventually be called "Severe Acute Respiratory Syndrome" (SARS). The Chinese government did not report the outbreak to the World Health Organization (WHO) for five months, during which time SARS spread through China to Taiwan, Hong Kong, Singapore, Vietnam, Thailand, Canada, and the United States. Eventually, in March 2003, an Italian infectious disease specialist, Dr. Carlo Urbani, alerted the world to the outbreak after he became infected while attending a medical conference in Thailand. The WHO subsequently recognized SARS and organized a global response to the developing pandemic. Before SARS was contained in July 2003, 8000 people from 29 countries had been infected and 774 died from SARS pneumonia, including Dr. Urbani.

We learned that SARS was a bat coronavirus originally transmitted to humans at Chinese "wet markets" where exotic animals such as pangolins (some of which were later proven to be infected with SARS) were sold for human consumption. SARS was highly contagious from patients to healthcare workers. Early in the outbreak, a third of reported cases were Chinese healthcare workers exposed in the line of duty. In March 2003, the admission of a single patient with SARS to a hospital in Hong Kong led to the infection of 99 hospital workers. A quarter of the ICU doctors working there eventually ended up on mechanical ventilators due to severe SARS pneumonia. I followed these events in 2002 with alarm and even began formulating a plan to quarantine our ICU staff in the hospital call rooms so we could work through a pandemic surge without the risk of bringing SARS home to our families. But by God's grace, SARS never established a strong foothold in the United States.

Research showed that certain medical procedures posed a high risk of transmitting SARS to healthcare workers. These included the use of high-pressure oxygen masks and endotracheal intubation (placing a breathing tube down the patient's throat to connect them to a mechanical ventilator). These methods would later be essential to the treatment of *Covid* pneumonia, but they are hazardous for healthcare workers because they aerosolize viruses from the patient's breath into the atmosphere. Fortunately, it was found that healthcare workers were protected from SARS by personal protective equipment (PPE) such as N95* facemasks, gowns and gloves. These findings were later used by the Centers for Disease Control (CDC) to develop infection control procedures for Covid. [*N95 masks are more protective than standard surgical masks, filtering out 95% of tiny airborne particles that convey* *viruses.*]

Eighteen years later, in early January 2020, the world learned of another outbreak of coronavirus pneumonia in China. The first cases occurred in November 2019 in close proximity to another wet market and the Wuhan Institute of Virology. This geographic association fueled competing theories that Covid was either transmitted from an animal vector (as SARS was) or by an accidental breach of containment at the Wuhan Institute of Virology, where potentially dangerous research into bat coronaviruses was conducted.

During the early stages of the outbreak, the number of cases doubled weekly in Wuhan and a Chinese ophthalmologist, Dr. Li Wenliang, surmised that an outbreak of SARS was occurring. He warned his colleagues to take precautions but was silenced by Chinese authorities. However, evidence of the outbreak soon became undeniable and the Chinese government reported it to the World Health Organization on December 31, 2019. By the end of January, Covid had spread to Thailand, Japan, Vietnam, South Korea, Germany, and the United States, and the WHO issued a global health emergency. On February 11, 2020, the WHO named the illness "Coronavirus Disease 2019" (COVID–19) after it had been determined that the cause was a coronavirus similar to the one that caused SARS.

I had previous occasions to worry about contagious infection exposure in my career, having taken care of many patients with advanced AIDS, tuberculosis and even Ebola. But I never felt threatened on a *daily* basis until after we saw our first case of Covid in February 2020 – a drunken man who came to our ER with severe vomiting, briefly evaluated for ICU admission before recovering and being discharged. About a week later, we were notified that a Covid test performed at another healthcare facility resulted positively. One of my partners and 14 other healthcare workers had been inadvertently exposed to Covid without any protection against airborne pathogens and were quarantined for 21 days.

This event exposed two early mistakes by the CDC that put frontline healthcare workers at risk. 1) The CDC initially developed and distributed a defective Covid test for use in the United States and had to recall it and go back to the drawing board. By March 2020, new more-reliable test kits were finally made available, but in short supply, completely inadequate for the explosive spread of Covid. So, *routine* testing of all patients, which would have prevented this exposure, could not yet be recommended. 2) The CDC originally recommended *against* universal masking in the hospital. Masking and Covid testing were only to be used for febrile pneumonia patients who had recent travel to areas in which Covid was rampant (i.e., China, Italy and Iran) or who had direct contact with a *confirmed* Covid case. This recommendation disregarded the possibility that the person-to-person spread of undiagnosed Covid could occur in the United States – something that we knew was inevitable and likely already happening at an accelerating pace.

As private-practice physicians, my partners and I were free to manage our own PPE, so I bought a case of N95 masks on eBay (at an incredibly marked-up price) and wore them whenever I thought a patient was suspicious. But our hospital policy, based on CDC recommendations, was binding for our nurses. When I saw patients with pneumonia of unknown cause who didn't meet CDC criteria for masking or testing, I could wear my N95, but the nurses couldn't. I felt ashamed whenever this happened, but failed to convince our administration to act contrary to CDC recommendations. Meanwhile, it was reported that over 3300 Chinese healthcare workers had been infected with Covid in the line of duty and that Dr. Li and five of his physician colleagues at Wuhan Hospital had succumbed to Covid pneumonia. The CDC finally loosened the criteria for masking and testing by the end of February 2020.

In March 2020, the WHO officially (and somewhat anti-climactically) declared Covid a pandemic. By this time, Covid was being reported from over 100 countries and was already exponentially spreading across parts of the United States. A large Covid outbreak occurred in a skilled nursing facility in King County, Washington demonstrating the inadequacy of our *standard* infection control procedures. One hundred one residents, 50 healthcare workers and seventeen visitors contracted Covid by person-to-person spread within the facility, which could be traced back to a single index patient. Half of the infected healthcare workers were hospitalized and 34 of the residents died from Covid pneumonia.

New York State reported its first confirmed Covid case on March 1: a 39-year-old healthcare worker. Epidemiologists later projected that there were probably already 10,000 cases of *undiagnosed* Covid in New York at that point, given how fast Covid spread thereafter. This was another proof of the inadequacy of the initial CDC testing recommendations. Within three weeks, over 10,000 *confirmed* cases and 129 deaths were reported and NYC Mayor De Blasio emergently requested 15,000 ventilators and 50 million sets of PPE (personal protective equipment: masks, gowns, gloves and face shields) from federal stockpiles as Covid cases doubled every three days and the healthcare system was overwhelmed. By the end of March, 77,000 Covid cases and 2,700 Covid deaths had occurred in New York State. In response, 76,000 healthcare workers from all across the United States traveled to New York, putting themselves in harm's way to shore up the trenches.

The global experience taught us a few things about Covid pneumonia before it reached Arizona in force. Patients with Covid presented with symptoms similar to influenza: cough, fever, headache, and body aches – some with nausea and diarrhea. One unusual symptom – anosmia (the loss of sense of smell) – was later found to be caused by virus invasion of the olfactory bulbs of the brain. Some people with Covid had no symptoms at all but were avidly contagious. This was a key difference between SARS and Covid – patients with SARS got sick *before* they became infectious and therefore isolation of symptomatic patients could block transmission. Covid patients were infectious *before* they got sick; isolation of sick patients was prudent but often too late. It was helpful, but could never completely halt transmission. On average, every patient with Covid infected two other people.

In serious cases, Covid caused *pneumonia*, in which the microscopic air-sacs ("alveoli") of the lungs became infected and filled up with pus as the immune system counterattacked. As this process worsened over about a week or so, the patient became short of breath and their lungs became unable to fully oxygenate their blood. Low blood oxygen can be measured by the patient's oxygen saturation (O2 sat) and an O2 sat below 92% indicated the need for hospitalization to administer oxygen. This happened in about one in ten cases of Covid pneumonia.

Pneumonia can be detected by chest X-ray, as you can see in the figures below. The first chest X-ray is normal: the lungs look black (the color of air on a chest X-ray) and the borders of the lungs are sharply defined. The second X-ray shows severe Covid pneumonia with fuzzy areas of whiteness in both lungs obscuring the borders, corresponding to areas of the lung filled with pus (fluid and white blood cells trying to fight off the infection). You don't have to be a radiologist to understand that the person with the second chest X-ray would have a very hard time breathing – they are essentially drowning.

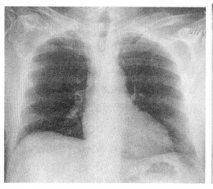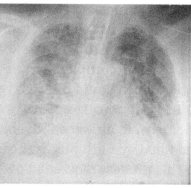

About one in twenty Covid patients developed *severe pneumonia**, requiring transfer to the ICU for high-pressure oxygen delivery via one of several devices. A high-flow nasal cannula is a device with tubing that can shoot a liter per second of 100% oxygen down a patient's nose! An even *more* powerful but less comfortable option, called "BiPAP" (Bilevel Positive Airway Pressure) requires a tight-fitting face mask that forces oxygen into the patient's nose and mouth under high pressure to assist their breathing. Unfortunately, both of these devices aerosolize the patient's exhaled breath into the atmosphere of their hospital room, increasing the chances that anyone in the room will be exposed to airborne Covid virus. [*This statistic and others quoted in this section, were published early in the pandemic when diagnostic testing was restricted and asymptomatic Covid cases went largely uncounted. This had the effect of somewhat inflating the perceived severity of Covid early in the pandemic.*]

The worst cases of Covid pneumonia required placement of an endotracheal tube or "ETT" to connect the patient to a mechanical ventilator. This required a physician to deeply sedate the patient and place an approximately one-foot-long ETT through the patient's mouth and down their throat into the trachea (the part of the throat leading to the lungs). Hence the term "endotracheal intubation" (or just "intubation"). During intubation, the physician looks straight down the patient's throat at close range, risking maximal exposure to Covid virus residing in the patient's lungs and throat. The ETT allows the patient to be connected to a mechanical ventilator, which uses pressurized oxygen to virtually take over the patient's breathing. If Covid continued to progressively damage the lungs, the amount of oxygen delivered by the ventilator was increased until it reached 100%*. The *pressure* required to fill the lungs also progressively increases until it is so high that the lungs may begin to rupture. [*Note that the O2 sat and oxygen delivery are confusingly both expressed as percentages but have opposite implications. The worse pneumonia gets, the lower the O2 sat will fall and the higher the required oxygen delivery will rise. Increasing oxygen delivery is used to keep the O2 sat around 90%, if possible, no matter how bad pneumonia gets.*]

One in fifty patients with a confirmed infection by early strains of Covid died, almost always from progressive pneumonia – making the Covid alpha strain about 20 times more lethal than H1N1 influenza. I had been an ICU doctor for 35 years but had never seen an organism even remotely this contagious *and lethal* at the same time. I moved into our guest bedroom at home, quarantining myself to avoid what seemed the eventuality of bringing Covid home to my wife and son.

One late night as I lay alone in our guestroom bed, unable to sleep due to anxiety, I remembered a patient I had seen more than twenty years before, during my fellowship training. I was sitting by his deathbed in the hospital, holding his hand as his pulse slowed; he commended his soul to God and recited Psalm 23 from memory. In the ensuing weeks, I was inspired to memorize Psalm 23, but as I lay sleepless in bed that night, I couldn't remember the words anymore. I pulled out my underutilized Bible and looked up Psalm 23. Over the next several nights, I practiced it whenever I lay awake. That helped.

The idea occurred to me to make a personal commitment

to prayer. I resolved to pray for a hundred consecutive days, which at the time seemed a lofty goal. I realized a great advantage – I had been a part-time member of a Bible study for some years, a bunch of great Christian men who would encourage and hold me accountable. I promised them I would text them a prayer a day for the next hundred days.

The prayers had to be short enough to comprise a reasonable-length text. I started with Psalms, then progressively searched other books of the Old and New Testaments for passages that stirred my soul, asking God's permission and guidance to rephrase them as relevant prayers. I included a few prayers from Dr. Martin Luther King Jr. and a few provided by my Bible study brothers, which I have properly attributed. Other prayers were completely original, born of listening to the Spirit, an ability that got stronger with practice.

Things got materially much worse in the days that followed. The global economy faltered, losing 34% of its stock value in little over a month. Our blind trust in the great American supply chain broke and even a simple trip to the grocery store became stressful and competitive. Our country seemed to be coming apart at the seams along racial and political rifts. A huge wildfire raged northeast of Phoenix, turning the sky an unnatural foreboding umber. By June 2020, the Covid hospitalization rate was higher in Arizona than in any other state or country in the world. The Navajo and other Native American people in Arizona were devastated by Covid.

In the ICU, we waged war against fear, dehumanization and exhaustion and it became clear that 100 days of prayer wouldn't be nearly enough. We battled hopelessness that winter as we witnessed the deaths of hundreds of Covid pneumonia patients despite the highest levels of life support we could provide. And when we finally thought the worst was behind us, the fall of 2021 became a battle against frustration as hundreds of patients who had refused vaccination again overflowed our ICU beds, some clinging to their belief Covid was a hoax even as they died from it. Although it was abundantly clear that the need for prayer would *never* be satisfied, enough important things had transpired that it seemed worth completing a record of them.

I was an eyewitness for the most part to the following stories. In some cases, the follow-up events are based on second-hand reports. Of course, the names, ages, gender, dates of hospital service, and a few other details have been changed to protect patient confidentiality. I have replaced some of my photographs with drawings for the same reason. Please honor my attempts to maintain privacy if you happen to have first-hand knowledge of these events – that is, please don't reveal the identity of the people described herein, *including me*.

I sincerely hope that my depiction of Native Americans involved in this story accurately conveys the respect with which I regard these great people.

Jesus said: "Do not be anxious about your life – what you will eat, nor about your body – what you will put on. For life is more than food, and the body more than clothing. Consider the ravens: they neither sow nor reap, they have neither storehouses or barns and yet God feeds them. Of how much more value are you than the birds! And which of you by being anxious can add a single hour to his span of life? If then you are not able to do as small a thing as that, why are you anxious about the rest?" [Luke 12:25]

"Ask, and it shall be given you; seek, and you shall find; knock, and it will be opened to you. For everyone who asks receives, and the one who seeks finds, and to the one who knocks it will be opened. Or which of you, if his son asks for a fish, will give him a serpent? If you then, who are evil, know how to give good gifts to your children, how much more will your Father who is in Heaven give good things to those who ask him?" [Matthew 7:10]

"Our Father, who art in Heaven, hallowed be thy name. Thy kingdom come, thy will be done on Earth as it is in Heaven. Give us this day our daily bread. Forgive us our trespasses as we forgive those who trespass against us. Lead us not into temptation but deliver us from evil." [Jesus's instruction on how to pray, circa 30 AD]

SPRING 2020: COURAGE

Prayer 1 (March 20, 2020)
The Lord is my shepherd I shall not want.
He makes me lie down in green pastures.
He leads me beside quiet waters.
He restores my soul.
He guides me in paths of righteousness for his name's sake.
Even though I walk through the valley of the shadow of death, I
shall fear no evil.
Your rod and your staff comfort me.
You prepare a feast for me in the midst of adversity.
You anoint my head with oil – my cup overflows.
Surely goodness and mercy will follow me all the days of my life
and I will dwell in the house of the Lord forever.

Driving into work at 5:30 am, the world had an eerie post-apocalyptic feel, the freeway and surface streets almost completely deserted due to the shutdown imposed by Arizona's Governor Doug Ducey. Schools were closed. Bars, movie theaters, gyms, dine-in restaurants, and all other non-essential businesses shut down. There was an executive decree that Arizonans stay at home except to carry out essential functions like grocery shopping and healthcare appointments. All elective surgeries in the state were canceled to free up hospital capacity for the anticipated surge of Covid pneumonia patients. But we had seen only a handful of Covid patients at our hospital so far. Besides the deserted feeling of the city all around us, it was a pretty typical day on-call in the ICU.

I stopped in for breakfast at the hospital cafeteria grill at about 6 am, as per my routine. Yuri was on grill duty, as he almost invariably was whenever I worked. Yuri was Armenian, super friendly, and outspoken. He had his own side business as a photographer and probably worked about 100 hours/week if you added it all up, but he had expenses – a wife, and *eight kids*.

"Doctor! – the usual?"

"Hey, Yuri. Yep, the usual – *an English muffin sandwich with one fried egg, ham, cheddar, and green chilis.* Don't you ever get a day off? I don't think I ever came in here when you weren't working!" I hated to think about when Yuri's last day off was.

"Someone called in sick, so I came in" he shrugged, *no big deal.* He turned to face the grill, getting to work with an industrial stainless steel spatula in each hand. He had about eight breakfasts going at the same time – chop, chop, chop, chop, bang, bang, bang, scrape scrape, scrape (cleaning his grill) – it was like an Armenian Benihanas.

The guy behind me in line ordered biscuits and gravy. Yuri scooped the gravy generously as always, but the guy looked unimpressed at his serving and said, "more."

"You want *MORE* gravy?" Yuri ladled about a quart more gravy over the biscuits, essentially drowning them. "I'll give you a bucket of gravy!" *Yuri was a great guy, but you didn't want to question how he made your food.*

I headed up to the hospital's third-floor ICU and printed up our patient list – eighteen patients – about average. They ranged in age from a 26-year-old man found down from a drug overdose to an 88-year-old woman with pneumonia. Three patients were in the unit with acute strokes and one with a heart attack. Two were transferred up from the floor with severe alcohol withdrawal – "delirium tremens" – a state of severe agitated confusion requiring intravenous sedation drugs. A smattering of the other usual cases: a patient with a ruptured aortic aneurysm, another with glioblastoma (cancer) of the brain, and another with alcoholic cirrhosis throwing-up blood. I would take care of half these patients today, plus any new patients being admitted.

Dr. Mayfield showed up, and together we took check out from Dr. Joyce, who worked nights for our group. Mayfield, Joyce, and I have known each other for most of our professional careers. I liked and respected them and hoped the feelings were mutual.

It took Joyce about twenty minutes to run through the patient list and fill us in on everything that happened overnight. Then she took off home to get some sleep. I would see her in twelve hours when I checked out to her on daytime events. *I was already looking forward to that.* Mayfield and I split up the patient assignments and got to work.

My normal routine was to review a few patients' computer records before going to the bedside to meet them – that way, I wouldn't look completely uninformed if they asked for test results. Chipping through the list that way would make for an easy day if it weren't for the almost constant interruptions: pages, phone calls, nurses tapping me on the shoulder, new admissions, and rounds. Sometimes while answering a page, I was paged two or three more times, giving me the impression that I could almost do a full-time job page answering – *God, I hated that pager!* Over the course of the day, I admitted patients with a pulmonary embolism (a blood clot in the lungs), a bacterial bloodstream infection from an impacted kidney stone, a subdural hematoma (a blood clot compressing the brain), and diabetic acidosis (a life-threatening complication of diabetes caused by insufficient insulin).

The last of my new patients, Elsie, was an 88-year-old woman transferred from the general hospital ward. She had been admitted from a nursing home with pneumonia three days earlier. A throat swab for influenza was negative. Antibiotics were started, although the cultures of her sputum didn't show bacterial pneumonia. As I stood at the computer terminal checking her labs and chest X-ray, I could hear a nurse persistently coughing down the hall. *How could she come into work with a cough?*

I peered in through the open door of Elsie's room. She was getting oxygen through a high-flow nasal cannula and coughing incessantly. We didn't know the etiology of Elsie's pneumonia, but whatever it was, it had to be airborne in her room. It struck me as strange to think at the time, but except for patients with tuberculosis and influenza, I never before thought twice about entering the room of a coughing patient without a mask. I ran back to my locker and put on one of my eBay N95s.

I washed my hands and donned a pair of blue nitrile gloves (standard infection control procedure) before entering Elsie's room to examine her. She was somnolent but seemed to be holding her own with her breathing. Her nurse Samantha entered the room unmasked to test Elsie's blood sugar. Sam came to the bedside and leaned right over Elsie to scan her wristband, their faces no more than 18 inches apart. Elsie was too sick to be trusted to cover her mouth if she suddenly coughed.

"Sam, you shouldn't be in here without a mask!"

"Oh, sorry, Dr. Eckshar, – um – but we aren't allowed to wear masks unless the patient is being tested for Covid."

"I'm wearing a mask because I'm not sure Elsie *doesn't* have Covid. You should too. You shouldn't be coming in here unprotected – she's coughing!"

"Well, *if* you order a Covid test, then we are allowed to wear a mask."

"I'm ordering the test! – just have to figure out what-all hoops to jump through to get the darn thing. Please just go get a mask!"

So the day went. Before I knew it, 7 pm had rolled around, and I realized I was tired and hungry. Thank God Joyce was here to cover the night. The traffic wouldn't be too bad; I could get home by 8 pm. I called my wife Jean on the way home, as was our custom, taking advantage of the drive time to catch up. Jean generally let me vent workplace frustrations for most of my half-hour commute. She was a grade school teacher but had picked up a lot of medicine over the past 35 years.

Prayer 2 (March 21, 2020)
Thank you Lord for your loving-kindness for choosing us to be your

sons and daughters. Help us to act as your children should.
Protect us and provide for us today.

News of China's Covid response depicted a cooperative, universally masked populace and immaculate healthcare facilities with no visitation allowed. The Covid wards looked like the sickbay from Star Trek, brave frontline healthcare workers protected head-to-toe in whole-body Tyvek suits.

The reality was very different in the United States. The CDC still hadn't recommended universal masking in our hospitals, although it was obvious that Covid was spreading fast, and there was no practical way to identify contagious patients, some of whom were asymptomatic. One local hospital system coined the condescending term "social comfort masking" – allowing nurses and doctors to wear their own masks at work while implying it was a psychological crutch rather than a prudent infection control strategy. One high-ranking MD administrator ridiculously warned that although social comfort masking was allowed, it could potentially lead to "self inoculation" – implying a person could catch Covid from themselves! *What medical school did they graduate from?*

The CDC should have admitted universal masking was prudent, but we just didn't have enough masks to do it. Instead, they pretended it wasn't necessary. I would like to have invited these policy-makers into the rooms of coughing pneumonia patients with me and ask them if they wanted to wear a mask or not.

Prayer 3 (March 22, 2020)
Jesus, we thank you for your sacrifice on our behalf.
We love you and worship you and ask that you continue to bless us.
Please keep our families safe and help us to use each day to advance your kingdom.
You did not spare your only Son, but gave him up for us all; how could we think now that you and he will not graciously give us all good things?
Help us to step out without fear today Lord, knowing you made

this great promise. We praise your holy name.
[Based on Romans 8:32].

I was CC'd this email sent from a frustrated frontline critical care physician to their hospital administrator: "In one of the most vivid scenes in the HBO miniseries 'Chernobyl', soldiers dressed in leather smocks ran out into a radioactive blast zone to shovel away fragments of the nuclear reactor core after it melted down. Here I am, working in a hospital in the most economically-advanced country in the world, being asked to fashion my own facemask out of cloth. Yesterday, I ran to the bedside of a crashing patient who might have Covid with two nurses and two respiratory techs. That's five N95 masks, gowns, face shields, and pairs of gloves for one patient. I saw 20 other patients that shift. If we are going to have to ration PPE, what percentage of those patients should I wear PPE for? The only reason the CDC is not recommending universal masking yet is that our country was unprepared and unwilling to retool and supply the safety equipment we need. The CDC's failure to recommend universal masking keeps healthcare workers at work without regard for our safety or that of our families. Giving healthcare workers the OK to wear bandanas for their 'social comfort' is like sending soldiers into battle wearing flip-flops."

Prayer 4 (March 23, 2020)
We have brought difficult days upon ourselves Lord, but let your loving-kindness and mercy abound all the more.
Build our faith in adversity Lord, like a rock against which no storm can harm us.

The first endotracheal intubation of a suspected Covid patient in our ICU was performed at 6:30 am by Dr. Joyce, right at the end of her 12-hour overnight shift. When I arrived for work, I found Joyce in a Covid isolation room, at the head of the bed, wearing an N95 mask *inside* an old "PAPR hood" (seen in the following photo). Needless to say, we didn't have

Tyvek suits like Chinese healthcare workers. The nurses in the room were wearing a hodgepodge of inferior-quality PPE. The gowns weren't moisture-proof – you could see right through the shabby material. June, a respiratory therapist (RT) who could speak Mandarin, told us that the labels of the Chinese-manufactured gowns read "Not for medical use." I noticed one of the nurses in the room had no eye protection. I asked the nursing supervisor why four nurses were risking exposure when only one was necessary, and she said the nurses all volunteered "So they could get experience in caring for Covid patients" – the first of many incredible instances of bravery and dedication demonstrated by our nurses in the face of Covid. I watched from behind glass outside the room.

The patient's name was Mary Beth, a 62-year-old woman immunocompromised due to arthritis medication. One of her workmates called in sick with pneumonia a week earlier, and four days after that, Mary Beth came into our ER with a 102° fever, cough, and pneumonia on chest X-ray. She was admitted to a regular hospital ward with no special isolation precautions (no use of masks or gowns). Routine testing for typical causes of pneumonia, such as influenza, were all negative, but she had not yet been tested for Covid. The floor nurses took care of Mary Beth unmasked for three days. Overnight, her breathing became increasingly rapid and shallow, her blood oxygen saturation ("O2 sat") fell to 88%*, and she was now exhausted, lethargic, and drenched in sweat. [*O2 sats below 90% necessitate escalation of oxygen therapy.]

Joyce immediately instituted full Covid precautions and transferred Mary Beth to the ICU for intubation and mechanical ventilation. Now, no one could enter Mary Beth's room without an N95 facemask, eye protection, gown, and gloves. Joyce sent off throat swab and sputum Covid tests, the full results of which wouldn't be reported until *after* Mary Beth left "the unit" (the ICU) five days later.

At the very end of their exhausting 12-hour shift, Joyce

and the night-crew nurses intubated Mary Beth, exposing themselves in the most intimate way to whatever micro-organism was causing her pneumonia. I respected their courage and was secretly relieved; they could have easily stalled 30 minutes and handed the intubation off to the daytime crew and me. I wondered at the time if I would have been as brave as they were.

March 23, 2020: *Joyce, intubating our first suspected Covid patient while wearing a positive airway pressure respirator (PAPR) hood – a reusable vinyl hood attached to a battery-powered air pump worn at the waist. These well-worn hoods were previously used by our environmental services department to train in responding to chemical spills. PAPR hoods were impractical for repeated every day use in the ICU, and there was no way to sterilize them effectively between users. Joyce swore she would never wear one again since she could neither hear nor be heard while she was wearing it.*

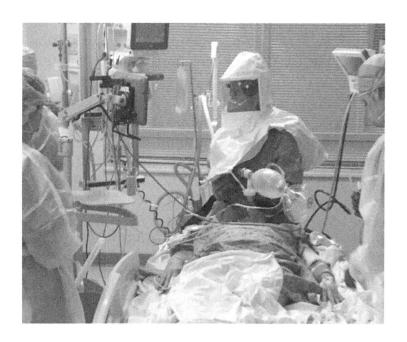

Prayer 5 (March 24, 2020)
Preserve me O God, for in you I take refuge.
I say to the Lord "You are my Lord, I have no good apart from you."
[Psalm 16 abbreviated]

We were awaiting the results of Covid testing on six other pneumonia patients besides Mary Beth.

Prayer 6 (March 25, 2020)
The Lord is a stronghold in times of trouble and those who know your name put their trust in you, O Lord, for you have not forsaken those who seek you.
Lord, thank you for our daily bread.
You give today's bread for today; help me not worry about tomorrow, trusting you will answer my prayer anew each day.

Prayer 7 (March 26, 2020)
I'm not proud of how I felt today Lord.
Only by your mercy am I saved and given a fresh chance to try again tomorrow.
Please protect us from Covid again today Lord – keep us safe here at work, and protect our homes and our families.

My first experience with Covid-anger: a young man had been found unconscious from a drug overdose at a crowded methamphetamine party house about a week ago, having of course ignored the statewide Covid lockdown. About a dozen of my colleagues took care of him without masking, as per hospital policy, when he was transported to our emergency room by EMS (emergency medical service). Today, we were informed that a Covid test, obtained on him several days earlier at *another* ER, had resulted positive. The entire team of healthcare workers had to be pulled out of the rotation and quarantined. They could theoretically already have been contagious to their families by the time the exposure was revealed. At least one, and possibly three, nurses caught Covid from this patient exposure. [*The exact outcomes of workplace*

Covid exposures were often hard to establish accurately. Official reports and personal accounts of nurses and other healthcare workers were sometimes contradictory.]

Prayer 8 (March 27, 2020)
Heavenly Father, your name is holy and your word is law in Heaven and on Earth.
Thank you for making us your children and forgiving our sins first.
Now we are mindful to forgive each other.
Keep your mighty arms around us.
[A partial version of "The Lord's Prayer"]

New York City was fast becoming the epicenter of the Covid pandemic in the United States, and its healthcare system, among the best-equipped in the world, was being overwhelmed. Covid was doubling in NYC every three days. A high percentage of patients became critically ill, each requiring weeks of life support. The state healthcare system had access to about 12,000 ventilators, but most were already in use. On March 26, Governor Cuomo officially approved the practice of "splitting mechanical ventilators" – hooking two patients up to the same life support machine! It's hard to overstate how crazy and desperate this sounded to those of us familiar with the normal operation of mechanical ventilators – like being on a sinking ship and being told to share your life vest. If this is what Covid was doing in NYC, the heart of our country's most advanced healthcare infrastructure, *what would happen when it hit rural Arizona?*

Prayer 9 (March 28, 2020)
Lord, we thank you for your mercy and sacrifice.
Please continue to watch over and protect us and our families.
Let this time be a time of home reunion and help those of us who venture out be a beacon of light, bringing others to your Kingdom.
We put our faith in you and thank you for letting us take part in your work. In your heavenly name, we pray.

Mary Beth was successfully "extubated" (the ETT

disconnected from the ventilator and removed from her throat) and transferred out to the floor. Both her Covid tests came back negative shortly afterward. Her quick recovery should have been a clue that she didn't have Covid pneumonia, but we didn't have enough experience at the time to know that.

Prayer 10 (March 29, 2020)
I bless the Lord who gives me counsel; in the night also my heart instructs me; because he is at my right hand, I shall not be shaken. Therefore my heart is glad and my whole being rejoices, my flesh also dwells secure, for you will not abandon me.
[Psalm 16 abbreviated]

All hospital-based doctors and nurses undergo mandatory annual training in the proper use of personal protective equipment (PPE) so that we can safely care for the occasional contagious patient. I had never before been so motivated to adhere to every detail of the proper procedure. I studied the CDC procedure for "donning and duffing Covid PPE," which consisted of 34 steps described in 18 online videos (not exaggerating!) These were just the 18 steps for duffing (taking off) PPE:

1) enter the duffing area,
2) disinfect outer gloves,
3) remove and discard outer gloves,
4) inspect and disinfect inner gloves,
5) remove the face shield,
6) disinfect inner gloves,
7) remove the coverall,
8) disinfect inner gloves,
9) remove boot covers,
10) change inner gloves,
11) remove/discard the N95*,
12) disinfect the new inner gloves,
13) disinfect your shoes,
14) disinfect inner gloves,
15) remove/discard inner gloves,

16) perform hand hygiene,
17) review for contaminants,
18) exit the duffing area.

You can imagine how impractical it would be to incorporate these CDC procedures into the workflow every time you entered/exited a Covid patient's room.

[*The outside of the N95 mask was considered contaminated, necessitating the mask be discarded after each use. But the hospital was only providing us one N95 mask per day – if we threw it away after the first use, what were we supposed to do the rest of the day?]

Prayer 11 (March 30, 2020)
Almighty Lord of all creation, my holy Father, I praise you and thank you for your endless patience and mercy.
Lord, humble me within, but make me strong in your Holy Spirit.
Bless my brothers and our families in these hard days, especially those whose livelihood and security are threatened.
Keep them safe and secure under your roof.

Prayer 12 (March 31, 2020)
Lord, every day of our lives is a gift from you, a chance to love and serve each other as you showed us, and to enjoy the beauty of this Earth you made for our temporary home.
Lord help us get the most out of this day.
Provide for us and protect us from evil.
[A derivation of the Lord's prayer]

The code bells went off on the hospital intercom system. *Ping! Ping! Ping! Ping!* My heart rate and blood pressure shot up as adrenaline flooded my bloodstream, awaiting the location announcement.

"Code blue room 558. Code blue room 558. Code blue room 558."

I jogged down the hall to the elevators – *alright, more of a brisk walk, my code-running days long past* – and got on with three of the code nurses, Samantha, Lynn, and Isaiah. We were silent, probably each taking personal stock. I prayed silently – inarticulate thoughts that might translate: *God grant that I do my job well – that the patient will not die because of my shortcomings.* Perhaps a self-centered prayer; the outcome of this code was not likely dependent on my performance.

Out of the elevator and down the hall, room 558 was easily identifiable by the crowd outside the door looking in. I grabbed a pair of large blue nitrile gloves as I entered the room, the only PPE provided.

Chaos in the room – staff milling around – a buzz of excited conversation. I pushed past some nurses to my station behind the head of the bed. My heart sank. The patient looked dead already. A man in his late 30's, probably close to 400 lbs. The hue of his lips was a deathly purple, some vomit in his beard. A respiratory "code blue." Intubating him was liable to be hugely complicated by his body habitus, which would obscure the anatomy of his throat and make it mechanically difficult to inflate his lungs. If I couldn't intubate him, he would certainly die. He looked like he would almost certainly die no matter what I did. *Lord, please help me not fail this man.*

The nurse doing CPR seemed to be doing a good job; it's very hard to give effective chest compressions to a patient this big. She had her elbows locked and was thrusting from her waist, getting her entire torso into the fast and deep compressions.

I turned to the RT assembling emergency equipment immediately to my left, and said: "Let's bag him!" Bagging him meant tightly holding an "Ambu bag" mask over his nose and mouth and squeezing the attached bag to deliver pressurized oxygen down his throat – a type of temporary hand-operated ventilator used until the patient can be intubated.

I directly addressed Samantha, who was standing beside the big red code cart: "Sam, give epinephrine 1 milligram IV." Communication was greatly enhanced among members of our ICU code team, who knew each other by name and also knew each of our respective roles. "Lynn, get me my intubation stuff, would you? 7.5 ETT and the Mac-4 – and have someone call trauma anesthesia to back me up in case this doesn't fly" – *anticipating I might not be able to intubate him.*

Louder, to the room of strangers at large: "DOES ANYONE KNOW WHY THIS PATIENT IS IN THE HOSPITAL?" I didn't know the floor team, and I didn't know anything about the patient. It was difficult to get even the most rudimentary clinical information from the floor team during the chaos of a code. There were at least ten looky-loos packed into the room who weren't on the code team, shuffling around, shoulder to shoulder, gabbing with each other. Typical; none paid me any attention.

The patient was very hard to bag. Oxygen was hissing out all around the mask seal every time the RT squeezed the bag. His beard was slick with vomit preventing the mask from sealing – only a near-perfect seal would allow us to deliver oxygen to his lungs with sufficient pressure to inflate his huge chest. Oral secretions and emesis were getting all over my gloves, and I could feel wetness on the bare skin of my forearms. The way things were now, all we were doing was spraying his secretions into the room. I better intubate him quickly – *what was taking so long with my intubation equipment?* I glanced at Lynn, who seemed to almost have it all together.

"WHO IS THIS PATIENT'S NURSE?"

A young floor nurse caught my eye, "Me!"

"What is this guy here for?"

"Heart failure. He was supposed to go home today."

"Does he have pneumonia?"

She shrugged, "He was on antibiotics."

Lynn was back, handing over the ETT and the Mac-4 laryngoscope used to open and look down the throat to the vocal cords, to guide the ETT into the trachea – *to "intubate".* The moment of truth.

I pulled the bag mask away, scissored his teeth open with my forefinger and thumb, and inserted the stainless steel laryngoscope, shoving his tongue out of the way. The back of his throat was filled with vomit obscuring the view – I cleared it with the suction wand, catching a whiff of sour breath. I peered closer, then drew back, trying to get my 60-year-old eyes in focus – *should get myself a pair of reading glasses.*

Please, please, please . . . there! The vocal cords.

I pulled up on the patient's jaw with the laryngoscope to adjust the view, passed the ETT down the patient's throat, and saw it pass right through the vocal cords – the best way to be sure it was in the right place. Easier than anticipated – *thank you Lord.* We attached the Ambu bag to the ETT and manually ventilated his lungs with 100% oxygen. We got a pulse back about two minutes later, and once he was stabilized for transfer, we moved him down to "the unit" (a colloquial term for the ICU).

I have run hundreds of codes over the past 35 years and been sprayed with all kinds of patient secretions in the process, but I had rarely worn a mask or face shield. What if this patient had Covid? We all would have gotten it.

Prayer 13 (April 1, 2020)
The Heavens declare the glory of God and the sky above proclaims his handiwork. The fear of the Lord is clean; the rules of the Lord are true.
Declare me innocent from hidden faults. Keep back your servant from presumptuous sins; let them not have dominion over me! Then I shall be blameless.
Let the words of my mouth and the meditations of my heart be acceptable in your sight, O Lord, my rock and my redeemer.
[Psalm 19 abbreviated]

Although we had only admitted a few moderately-ill Covid patients to our hospital so far, increasing reports of outbreaks of Covid *within* healthcare facilities were heightening our sense of impending doom. In the spring of 2020, hand-to-mouth transmission from contaminated surfaces was thought to be an important mechanism in the spread of Covid. A study from Wuhan reported that Covid virus proteins were detectable on 43% of bedrails, 67% of the air ventilator ducts, 70% of floors, and 75% of computer mice in the ICU. Many of us worked out elaborate daily routines for decontaminating desktops, computer keyboards, and mouses in our workspaces. I washed my hands each time I touched a doorknob or other potentially contaminated surface, perhaps as many as 50 times in a 12-hour ICU shift. Luckily, we seemed to have ample supplies of alcohol-based hand sanitizer.

In early April, the CDC reported 50,000 confirmed cases of Covid in US healthcare workers – a rate three times higher than in the general population. The median age of those infected in the line of work was 42 years; 55% reported *only* workplace exposure, and 62% reported no underlying chronic illnesses.

Prayer 14 (April 2, 2020)
The Lord is my light and my salvation; whom shall I fear?
The Lord is the strength of my life; of whom shall I be afraid?
One thing only I have asked of the Lord, that I may dwell in the house of the Lord all the days of my life, to behold the beauty of the Lord, and to inquire in his temple.
For in the time of trouble, he shall hide me in his temple; he shall set me high on a rock. And now shall my head be lifted up.
[Derived from Psalm 27]

Prayer 15 (April 3, 2020)
My soul continually remembers my sin and is bowed-down within me. But this I call to mind, and therefore I have hope: The steadfast love of the Lord never ceases, his mercies never come to an end. They are new every morning.
Great is your faithfulness. The Lord is my portion says my soul; forevermore I will hope in him.
[Derived from Lamentations 3:20-24]

I learned on rounds (when our team of doctors, nurses, pharmacists, and various specialty therapists, walk around the unit discussing the plan for each patient) that one of our housecleaning staff had been hospitalized for Covid pneumonia. Cleaning ICU rooms is hazardous, entailing exposure to nearly every human body fluid that can be excreted or extracted by needle, all of which might accidentally get spilled or sprayed about the room at one point or another during a chaotic admission. Our housekeepers had not yet been provided masks.

Joyce called in sick later that morning. She had a 105° fever, a dry cough and an intense headache and body aches. She said she never felt so sick in her entire life. An ER chest X-ray showed pneumonia, and an influenza swab was negative, but Covid testing was not performed. Drive-through Covid testing sites were just opening in a few locations, but Joyce felt too sick to drive. Mayfield (previously quarantined for workplace Covid exposure back in February) finagled a Covid throat swab kit into his possession by questionable means and personally drove out to Joyce's house, donning full PPE to test her out on her driveway.

Prayer 16 (April 4, 2020)
In you, Lord my God, I put my trust.
Show me your ways Lord, teach me your paths.
Turn to me and be gracious.
Relieve the troubles of my heart.
Look upon my affliction.
Guard my life and rescue me, for I take refuge in you.
[Psalm 25 abbreviated]

Prayer 17 (April 5, 2020)
God my savior, guide me in your truth, for my hope lies with you alone. Remember, O Lord, your great mercy and love from times of old. Remember not my sins.
For your name's sake O Lord, forgive my iniquity, though it is great.
Turn to me and be gracious to me, for I am lonely and afflicted.
Look upon my distress and take away my sins!

[Continued, from Psalm 25]

There was no official guidance on how doctors and nurses exposed to Covid in the line of duty could protect their families at home, but this was one of my foremost concerns. The last thing I wanted to do was bring Covid home to Jean and our son.

I developed the following protocol: I wore hospital scrubs over my usual work clothes, tossing them in the hospital's dirty-laundry bins at the end of each shift. When I got home, I closed the garage door and took off my shoes, socks, and work clothes. The clothes went into a "contamination hamper" in the garage. My work shoes stayed in the garage overnight, never again entering our house – *a study had found Covid virus protein on 50% of ICU workers' shoes!* I then showered and put on clean clothes. Our guest bedroom/bath became my exclusive habitation. I slept alone. It goes without saying that I had to give up some of my worse eating habits (e.g., spooning ice cream straight out of the carton). I put a Purell dispenser next to our refrigerator but generally tried to simply never go in there. Jean made food for me on paper plates that I threw out after eating. [In retrospect, this was probably going overboard, but my thought at the time was that it was worthwhile to try as best I could to protect the ones I love.]

Prayer 18 (April 6, 2020)
The Lord is good to those who wait for him, to the soul who seeks him.
It is good that one should wait quietly for the salvation of the Lord.
Worthy are you, our Lord and God, to receive glory and honor and power, for you created all things, and only by your good will do they continue to exist.
Lord, first thing today, we look upon creation and say thank you. We ask that you not allow the worries of the world affect our position of praise and worship and joy in you.
Help us to put all things in your hands today.
Strengthen us to help and encourage our brothers and sisters.

Thank you Jesus, for this blessed day.
[Taken from Lamentations 3:20-26, and Revelations 4:11, offered by Mike U.]

Joyce's Covid result was negative. She recovered and returned to work two weeks later. A false alarm perhaps, but one I remained suspicious of, learning shortly thereafter that Covid tests provided false negative results in people infected with Covid 30% of the time.

Joyce's close call brought to mind my old friend Carlos, who was in his early 70s but still practicing critical care in Chicago, where Covid was beginning to surge. Back in the day, Carlos once bicycled across the entire continental US. But he had heart disease and emphysema now. Contemporaneous data from Italy (an early epicenter of the pandemic) suggested that the fatality rate among men of Carlos' age range infected with Covid might be as high as 20%; *odds worse than Russian roulette!* I decided I should call Carlos and be sure he weighed the risk he was taking at work. *Maybe it was time for him to retire.*

I called him. We caught up a little; I beat around the bush, then told him I thought he should consider retiring to protect himself. Carlos was touched that I would think of him, but the idea of quitting medicine was shocking to him – out of the question. He was a doctor! What would he do with himself if he wasn't taking care of patients?

Soon thereafter, Carlos was at the tip of the spear as Covid hammered Chicago. Later, when things there settled down, he flew out to Albuquerque, New Mexico, to help in an understaffed ICU during the peak of *their* Covid surge. Carlos is one of those doctors who will probably never get to retire but just go right on working 'til the day he dies. More about this great old-time physician later.

Prayer 19 (April 7, 2020)
I wanted to ask for prayer today for a patient named Joseph, who traveled here from Oregon seeking alternate therapy for

terminal cancer.

Lord God, thank you for bringing another brother into our midst.
We just met Joseph Lord, but you knew him and loved him from
before he was born. And you love his family, even more than he
does.
All power in Heaven and on Earth is yours Lord.
Say the word and Joseph will be healed.
Say the word and he will get on a plane and get home to Oregon.
Bless and strengthen his faith.
Bless and strengthen his family.
We call out as your children in the name of your son Jesus.
We love you and we trust you Lord Jesus!

Joseph boarded the outbound flight in Oregon under his own power but found he couldn't stand up when the plane landed at Sky Harbor. A cancer metastasis had compressed his spinal cord during the flight, leaving him paralyzed from the chest down. He required intubation shortly after being transported from the airport to our hospital. He was alert, had decent strength in his arms, and could communicate by showing us messages he typed on his cell phone (it being virtually impossible to speak with an ETT in place). But his legs were completely paralyzed, and his breathing muscles partially so. Imaging showed the spinal lesion was inoperable. Joseph was treated with dexamethasone (a potent steroid), but his prognosis was grim.

Prayer 20 (April 8, 2020)
He who dwells in the shelter of the Most High will rest in the
shadow of the Almighty.
I will say of the Lord: "He is my refuge and my fortress, my God in
whom I trust."
If you make the Most High your dwelling – even the Lord who is my
refuge – then no harm will befall you, no disaster will come near
your tent. For he will command his angels concerning you to guard

you in all your ways, and they will lift you up in their hands.
"Because he loves me," says the Lord, "I will rescue him; I will
protect him for he acknowledges my name. He will call upon me,
and I will answer him. I will be with him in trouble; with long life I
will satisfy him and show him my salvation."
[Joseph shared this prayer from Psalm 91]

Joseph *had* to get back home to his family, but the logistics of flying on a ventilator were practically insurmountable. Getting him *off* the ventilator would make things much easier, but he didn't seem strong enough to effectively cough and keep his windpipe clear. I was pretty sure that without an ETT, Joseph would choke to death on his own saliva.

However, he was insistent, and the next day after much debate and prayer, I extubated Joseph with trepidation. It was almost immediately apparent this was a mistake, as he began choking, unable to clear his throat. I put the palm of my hand on the pit of his stomach, shoving inward each time he tried to cough. Working together like this, the two of us were able to temporarily clear his windpipe. *But how was he going to do on his own?* The nurse and I watched over him closely that afternoon as he tenuously "hung in there."

Prayer 21 (April 9, 2020)
I fall to my knees and pray to the Father, the Creator of everything
in Heaven and on Earth.
I pray that from his glory, he will empower me with inner strength
through his Spirit. Then Christ will make his home in my heart and
I will trust in him.
My roots will grow down into God's love and keep me strong and I
will be granted the ability to grasp, as all God's people should, how
wide, how long, how high, and how deep his love is.
May I experience the love of Christ, though it is too great to
understand fully. Then I will be made complete with all the fullness
of life and power that comes from God through his son Jesus Christ.
[Derived from Ephesians 3:14-20]

Joseph made it through the night. He worked out a one-man cough-assist technique by pushing on the pit of his stomach with his hands. It was just enough to help his weakened diaphragm generate an effective cough. He made airline arrangements on his cellphone with a stubborn faith he would be able to keep it up long enough to make it home. He understood the risk and I didn't have the heart to stand in his way. I discharged him against my better medical judgment and said a prayer for his safe journey home.

Prayer 22 (April 10, 2020, Good Friday)
Jesus fell on his face and prayed, saying: "My Father, if it is possible, let this cup pass from me; nevertheless, not as I will, but as you will." And there appeared to him an angel from Heaven strengthening him. And being in agony he prayed more earnestly and his sweat became like great drops of blood falling to the ground.
Lord Jesus – you took all the shame and guilt and just punishment of my sins upon your blameless self and through your sacrifice, made me clean in your Father's eyes.
I remember your great suffering on my account this Good Friday.
[Taken from Luke 22:42-44]

Our first critically ill Covid patient was admitted on Apr 10, 2020. McKale was a previously healthy 45-year-old man of the Hopi nation. When asked how he had been exposed to Covid, he simply answered, "My whole family has it." McKale had been transferred down to us from an ER in Holbrook, Arizona, 170 miles away, as rural facilities in northern Arizona were being overrun by Covid. On arrival, McKale already required high-flow nasal cannula oxygen.

Prayer 23 (April 11, 2020)
Lord, all it says about this day in the Gospels is that,"On the Sabbath they rested according to the commandment." Thank you for the rest of the story.
We await the celebration of your resurrection with great hope: for

the empty tomb on Sunday morning, for our coming King, for the end of a worldwide pandemic, relief of our own personal suffering, and most of all, for your eternal kingdom that can never be shaken, no matter what darkness abides on Earth.

Help us put our worries aside and rest today in complete security, knowing your triumph and our salvation are assured.

We praise you and thank you Lord Jesus.

McKale had deteriorated to the point that he required intubation and Mayfield was prepared. He had built his own "intubation box" with MacGyver-like ingenuity – made of plexiglass sheets glued together with silicone to fit over McKale's head and neck. Two arm-holes had been cut through the front to admit the intubating physician's arms. Mayfield also spread a Home Depot painting tarp over McKale to help keep Covid-infected secretions out of the air. The intubation succeeded despite how clumsy the intubation box made things. It was a great idea in theory, but none of us ever used it again.

Later that day, Joseph texted me a picture of a pine sapling growing through the snow with two small branches one to a side, forming the shape of the cross – a picture taken that morning outside his home in Oregon. He had made it home.

Prayer 24 (April 12, Easter day)

Dear Lord, as we look out at this day help us to appreciate the life you gave us: Life here on Earth, and life in eternity with you.

Help us to remember how you sacrificed and emptied yourself to become one of us, to live the good life that we couldn't and to die the horrible death we deserved.

Help us to remember you did this to show your great love for us and to glorify your Father in Heaven.

Thank you for beating death and rising three days later.

This day is our greatest celebration! But help us remember to celebrate your victory every day, in good times and bad, as we are going through now.

You are our hope. You are our joy.

You are our king! Alleluia, He has risen!

I imagined the two Marys (Mary of Magdalene and Mary of Cleopas), whispering together before dawn, planning to go to Jesus's tomb early Easter morning: "The men are all asleep. Are you asleep?"

"No, I can't sleep."

"Do you want to go to the tomb?"

"Yes – let's go! Just the two of us!"

I don't know what they were expecting to find, but they probably never imagined that an angel and the risen Lord Jesus would appear to them.

McKale's O2 sat fell into the 80% range (dangerously low) despite receiving 100% oxygen at the highest ventilator pressure we could risk. The next best option was to try a proning bed (pictured below) – a bulky device used to turn him face-down (prone). This position improves the balance between blood flow and oxygen distribution in the lungs, improving the O2 sat of most patients with severe Covid, and potentially improving survival. Patients can be proned manually, but some outweigh our nurses by three or four-fold. Proning beds were worthwhile to prevent nursing injuries – *we didn't have any nurses to spare!*

The patient in this proning bed is in a face downward (prone) position, and is almost invisible – only a small portion of their right arm can be seen. The physical isolation of the patient imposed by the proning bed would later become a source of vicarious personal distress for everyone working in the unit, but at this   early point in the pandemic, it was still more of a novelty.

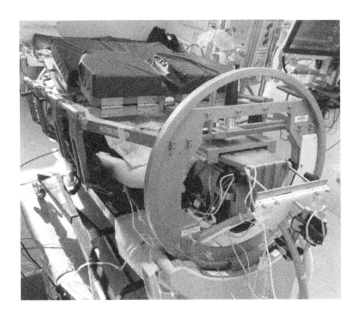

Prayer 25 (April 13, 2020)

As the deer pants for streams of water, so my soul pants for you my God.
These things I remember as I pour out my soul: how I used to go to the house of God under the protection of the Mighty One with shouts of joy and praise.
Why my soul are you so cast down?
Why so disturbed within me?
Put your hope in God, for I will yet praise him, my Savior and my God!
Deep calls to deep in the roar of your waterfalls; all your breakers have swept over me.

By day the Lord directs his love, and at night his song is with me.
[Taken from Psalm 42]

Seeing McKale in a proning bed dramatically changed my mindset towards his care and prognosis. I have to admit a personal fear of proning beds. They entomb the person within like a high-tech sarcophagus, rendering them completely helpless – unable to communicate, unable to move, except perhaps to twitch their fingers – their limbs and torso encased in high-density foam and locked inside the massive steel outer shell. If conscious, they experience severe sensory deprivation and disorientation – *who knows how the patient's delirious mind might interpret their situation?* Worse of all, proning is one of our final options, and as such, a concrete indication that the chances of patient survival have become diminishingly small.

Prayer 26 (April 14, 2020)
I waited patiently for the Lord; he inclined to me and heard my cry.
He drew me up from the pit of destruction and set my feet upon a rock. He put a new song in my mouth, a song of praise to our God.
Many will see and fear and put their trust in the Lord.
Walk with me dear Lord, so that I don't face this day alone.
Your presence is a like lighthouse shining in the darkness to lead me safely home. I pray that I will reflect the light of your loving-kindness to my brothers and sisters.
In the name of Christ, bless me and all whom I meet today.
[A modern interpretation of Psalm 40]

The unit depends on many support staff. Today as I was working on some charting, Marg from food services came into the ICU rolling a stainless-steel food rack filled with dozens of plastic patient food trays; the rack was almost as tall as she was. There were a few liter plastic jugs of khaki-colored tube feedings on top, *reminding me of when I was a starving resident on night call; I once slugged one of these down and can thereby testify they are not for oral consumption!*

I had seen Marg being dropped off in front of the hospital

a few times in the early morning – found out she didn't own a car, but had a reliable neighbor who drove her to and from work every day. She was Medicare-aged and had confided in me a time or two about some medical issues she was struggling with. She was essentially a poster child for Covid risk factors, unmasked and interacting with dozens, perhaps hundreds of sick people each day all over the hospital. A trooper, she kept her nose to the grindstone.

"Hey, Marg! Got anything good to eat in there? Sausage pizza?"

"Oh, Hi, Doctor! No, sorry, no pizza today!" she smiled, blushing. I silently prayed for her protection from Covid.

Prayer 27 (April 15, 2020)
Thank you Lord for blessing me and keeping me.
Thank you for making your face shine upon me and being gracious to me.
Thank you for lifting up your countenance upon me.
I pray today that you give me your peace. Peace in your love, and peace in your son, whom you have given so lovingly to save me.
Your grace abounds and gives me strength!
Thank you Lord Jesus, in your name I pray.
[Taken from Numbers 6:24-26]

McKale's life was hanging by a thread despite the highest level of life support we could provide. We wouldn't have any proven therapy for Covid until mid-June, nearly two months away. Hydroxychloroquine was being internationally touted in the lay press, but there were no reliable scientific studies to support its use*. (One Arizona man fatally overdosed himself ingesting chloroquine phosphate aquarium cleaner in an attempt to protect himself from Covid). We decided to try convalescent plasma – the fluid component of blood from patients who had recovered from Covid. Convalescent plasma contains anti-Covid antibodies, which might theoretically help fight off Covid pneumonia, but they could only be acquired through a research protocol. Throughout the coming months, we adhered to an important ethical principle of modern medicine: only therapies *proven* to be safe and effective should be given to patients by bedside doctors. Unproven therapies should only be given as part of formal research. This principle would be considerably challenged by desperation and misinformation as the pandemic progressed. [*Well-conducted clinical trials later proved that hydroxychloroquine did not effectively prevent or treat Covid.*]

Prayer 28 (April 16, 2020)
Lord, make me a man after your own heart.
Let me see your loving purpose in everything that happens whether it seems good or bad to me.
Give me a humble heart Lord, ears that can hear your words and take them to heart.
What is this block of concrete in my heart, Lord, holding back my faith? Say the word and heal me and make me what I am supposed to be, secure in the faith given me.
I praise your holy name!
["The Cinder Block Prayer"]

On this day, universal masking was *finally* allowed at our hospital and henceforth required for everyone coming in the door. Nurses and doctors were also routinely provided with a single N95 mask for each 12-hour shift to use when seeing Covid patients. N95 masks were contaminated after a single use and it would previously have been considered a serious breach of infection control procedures to carry a used mask around the hospital and repeatedly reuse it, but our infection control specialists were suddenly now *recommending* the practice. This wasn't at all reassuring to those of us behind the masks – we *knew* it was potentially unsafe, necessitated only by the sorry state of our PPE supplies.

Prayer 29 (April 17, 2020)
Thank you Lord for another day.
Your grace is sufficient for me. Let me hold onto you closer, grab

tighter and release my hold on these earthly things.
Let my heart seek you like a deer panting for water.
Help us all be laborers in your holy work.
You blessed us with this command: "Therefore do not be anxious about tomorrow, for tomorrow will be anxious for itself. Sufficient for the day is its own trouble." Please drive this into our hearts, Lord.
In Jesus's name, the name above all names, I pray.
[Prayer offered by Mike U. based on Matthew 6:34]

Prayer 30 (April 18, 2020)
I prayed for you to provide for me and my family last night Lord. Woke up refreshed. Your sun was rising behind your McDowell mountains with beautiful orange clouds on the horizon. Got to work safely. Had a good breakfast.
Every good thing I take for granted should be appreciated Lord.
Your miracles and loving-kindness are all-encompassing.
Many thanks Lord for the gifts of life, faith, salvation and family.

McKale's condition leveled out, then slowly began improving. We were able to supine him (turn him face-up) and take him out of the proning bed. This allowed Isaiah, his nurse, to clean him up. McKale had pressure sores over his nose, chin and cheeks, which we came to recognize as the stigmata of a proning bed survivor. But Mckale had been deeply sedated to tolerate proning and was still nearly comatose. It could take him a week to fully metabolize those sedation medications and wake up enough to begin breathing again on his own.

Prayer 31 (April 19, 2020)
Blessed is the man whom you discipline, O Lord, and whom you teach your law, to give him rest from days of trouble. When the cares of my heart are many, your consolations cheer my soul.
I have looked upon you in the sanctuary, beholding your power and glory. Because your steadfast love is better than life, my lips will praise you. So I will bless you as long as I live; in your name I will lift up my hands.

Oh Lord, please give us hearts of worship today!
[Taken from Psalms 94 and 63, offered by Mike U.]

Some of the things I concerned myself with early in the pandemic already seem a bit hard to understand in retrospect – *how could I have been thinking about T-shirts amid the developing catastrophe?* But I somehow got the idea that we needed T-shirts as a demonstration of solidarity within our ICU team. We worked through Custom Ink to have shirts made for ourselves and other team members, from nursing to housecleaning. Dr. Carlos bought over a hundred for the nurses in his hospital in Chicago. We put the money earned from T-shirt sales into a fund that our nurses could access to assist disadvantaged families of our ICU patients, but since visitation was soon halted, that money wasn't put to use right away. It comes back into the story about a year later in relation to three Covid orphans.

Our T-shirt logo: *Note the winged snakes of the Caduceus attacking the Coronavirus on top of the staff.*

COVID - 19 FRONTLINE CRITICAL CARE RESPONSE TEAM

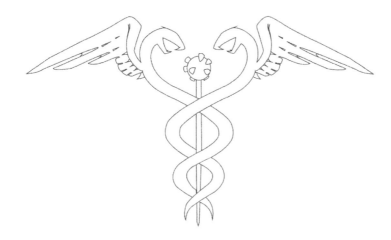

Prayer 32 (April 20, 2020)

Now our God, hear the prayers of your servant.

We do not make requests of you because we are righteous, but because of your great mercy.

Lord listen! Lord forgive! Lord, hear and act! For your sake, my God, do not delay, because your city and your people <u>bear your name</u>. [Taken from Daniel 9:4-19]

McKale continued to improve. He awoke and his ventilator was adjusted to allow him to begin progressively taking over his own breathing. This phase of his care focused on getting him off the ventilator before he developed secondary pneumonia with opportunistic bacteria, *a complication that would be the final nail in the coffin of many Covid patients we were to see in the coming months.*

Prayer 33 (April 21, 2020)

Will you not revive us again so that your people may rejoice in you? Show us your steadfast love, O Lord, and grant us your salvation.

Let me hear what God the Father says, for he will speak peace to his people. Surely his salvation is near to those who fear him, so that his glory may abide in our land.

Steadfast love and faithfulness meet; righteousness and peace kiss each other. Faithfulness springs up from the ground and righteousness looks down from the sky.

Yes, the Lord will give what is good and our land will yield its increase. Righteousness will go before him and we will follow in his footsteps. [From Psalm 85]

The Chief Medical Officer of our hospital bought thirty 3M "P100 full face respirator masks" for the ICU staff to wear when seeing Covid patients! This was the best protection money could buy (at least until Covid vaccine became available in mid-December 2020). This mask had an inch-wide silicone elastomer gasket that formed a tight seal around your whole face, nose and mouth. P100 filters remove 99.7% of relevant particles, making it virtually impenetrable if properly worn.

When putting a P100 on, we were careful to get all our hair out from under the forehead gasket, then block the exhalation valve with the palm of our hand while forcefully exhaling; the effort required to overcome the seal (and produce what sounded suspiciously like a fart) indicated whether the seal was adequate. P100s had a distinctive rubbery smell, and breathing through the dense filters was like breathing through a straw. But we got used to them over time and eventually could wear one for several hours at a time before having to take it off.

April 2020. *My 3M Full Face Respirator with P100 filters. I shaved off my beard to improve the seal. I could never put this mask on without immediately developing an itchy nose. Think of how scary it would be for a patient to meet a doctor decked out like this.*

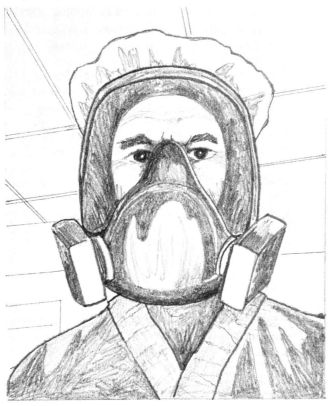

Prayer 34 (April 22, 2020)
Father, grant us courage like the Apostle Paul had through faith, so that not even the threat of death would frighten us.
For those of us you have chosen, death is not the loss of life, but being "swallowed by life" more abundant than we can imagine. Then we will leave these tattered old tents – our beat-up old bodies – and join you in your mansion. And the gift that meant the most to us here, our faith, will no longer be needed.
For we won't need to have faith anymore to believe in that which

we can plainly see.
[Taken from 2 Corinthians 5]

We had only two rooms in our ICU with negative pressure ventilation designed to contain airborne contagion, previously used for patients with tuberculosis. This obviously wasn't going to be enough space for Covid patients – *who would eventually come to fill up every bed in the entire ICU.* So we began cohorting our slowly increasing number of Covid patients in a separate area of the ICU, grouping them behind closed fire doors in an attempt to protect the other patients and staff from continuous exposure. We only entered the Covid cohort zone of the ICU when necessary for direct patient care.

Prayer 35 (April 23, 2020)
There is none like you, O Lord, nor are there any works like yours.
All nations shall come and worship before you Lord, and shall glorify your name, for you are great and do wondrous things.
You alone are God!
Teach me your way Lord, that I may walk in your truth. Train my heart to fear your name.
I give thanks to you, O Lord my God, with my whole heart and I will glorify your name forever.
[From Psalm 86]

I admitted a patient named Kira to the Covid cohort zone – a 44-year-old Navajo woman with no significant past medical history. She had severe Covid pneumonia but was very strong and able to hold her own for several days with the help of a high-pressure "BiPAP" mask that she could take off briefly to eat or drink. I had a gut feeling that she was going to do OK. I noticed she wore a crucifix and she readily accepted when I asked her if we could pray together.

"Lord Jesus – I know you were in this hospital room with Kira before I arrived and will stay with her long after I leave.
You knew her before she was born and you love her.
She is your daughter, and you are her Father, her protector.

Lord, you have all power in Heaven and Earth, and we know that what you say goes. Heal Kira! Make her stronger Lord.
Don't let her give up. Heal her lungs from this pneumonia Lord. Make her breathe strong again.
Get her back to her friends and family Lord –to her home where she belongs.
Say the word and it will happen.
We believe. We trust you and love you Lord Jesus!"

Prayer 36 (April 24, 2020)
Have mercy on me, O God, for I know my transgressions, and my sin is ever before me.
Against you only have I sinned, so that you may be justified in your judgment, but wash me and I will be whiter than snow.
Hide your face from my sins.
Create in me a clean heart, O God, and renew a right spirit within me, for you will not delight in sacrifice or I would give it.
The sacrifices of God are a broken spirit; a broken and contrite heart, O God, you will not despise!
[Psalm 51 abbreviated]

We were rounding outside the room of a newly admitted 52-year-old Covid pneumonia patient named George. His nurse said he was a jogger, a bit of a "fitness nut." A BiPAP mask was barely holding his O2 sat at 92%, but as we passed his room, he could be seen standing beside his bed, facing it with both hands on the mattress, jogging in place! His laptop was plugged-in on his bedside table and logged into CNN. Hopeful signs; he didn't seem apt to let Covid beat him. I never directly took care of George but made a point to look in on him henceforth each day when we passed his room on rounds.

Prayer 37 (April 25, 2020)
Lord Jesus. You are worthy of our trust – so worthy.
You are the hearer of prayers. The consoler of the suffering. The one whose slightest touch heals all disease.
We love you Lord. We thank you.

You do not disappoint the faithful.
All praise to you for being our shepherd in this valley of the shadow of death. All praise to you!

I went by to see McKale first thing this morning. His ventilator weaning had gone well; we had been able to steadily reduce his ventilator settings and allow him to gradually take over the work of breathing. I was optimistic we might soon be able to liberate him from the ventilator altogether. Extubation was one of my favorite job duties – it was almost like witnessing a birth when your patient takes their first free breath again after a brush with death; the most concrete milestone of ICU recovery. But I tried to temper my enthusiasm and act objectively, carefully running down the standard checklist of physiological parameters to assess McKale's readiness to breathe on his own. Everything looked copasetic. Next, the eyeball test. McKale looked washed-out but alert.

"McKale, do you want that breathing tube out?"

His brow furrowed a moment, then his eyes opened wide as it dawned on him that this was his chance to get rid of that plastic "garden hose" rammed down his throat, and he shook his head "yes" enthusiastically, waving his hands around for emphasis. *I secretly believe that how a patient answers this simple question may be more predictive than any of the objective physiological parameters on my checklist.* I asked Lynn's opinion – she was on board too. We gave McKale the good news and called the RT over to extubate.

"Pulling the tube" always took a lot longer than expected, and the process must seem interminable to an alert patient gagging on an ETT. June, the RT, set up suctioning equipment, oxygen delivery nasal prongs and an Ambu bag (in case things went south). The tape anchoring the ETT to McKale's face was gently pulled free using alcohol wipes to loosen the adhesive without tearing his fragile skin. Then June assiduously suctioned as deep as she could get down McKale's throat. A towel was placed on McKale's chest to receive the ETT. She warned him that she was going to make him cough as she deflated the ETT cuff (and whatever oral secretions remained spilled into his airway). Then she smoothly pulled the 30 cm long ETT and 100 cm nasogastric tube out and dropped them on the towel, which was then swaddled up and set aside. McKale scrunched up his face, experienced a paroxysm of coughing, then tried to weakly spit out the phlegm he brought up. June put the suction wand just to his lips so he could clear things out. Then McKale's face relaxed, his breathing slowed, and his throat cleared. June commanded him to open his mouth so she could suction him again, with which he begrudgingly complied. Then she put oxygen prongs in his nose; we sat him up straighter in bed, stood back and took a look at him. He looked OK. McKale was breathing on his own for the first time in almost two weeks!

It was with a great sense of achievement that I called to give his family the good news. But McKale's accomplishment was overshadowed by sorrow as we learned that McKale's grandmother, and two uncles had passed away from Covid during McKale's ICU stay.

Prayer 38 (April 26, 2020)
When I kept silent, my bones wasted away, for day and night your hand was heavy on me. Then I acknowledged my sin to you and did not hide my iniquity.
I said, "I confess my transgressions to the Lord." And you forgave my guilt through the blood of your son Jesus. Therefore I am counted among the faithful.
I pray to you while you may be found, and surely the rising of the mighty waters will not reach me.
You delight me with songs of deliverance.
You teach me the way to go – following Jesus' footsteps.
Your unfailing love surrounds me.
[Psalm 32 updated with the Good News, offered by Frank P.]

Kira's pneumonia worsened and she was being worn down by the progressively increasing work of breathing. The aid of the BiPAP mask was no longer sufficient. Kira assented with a curt nod when I recommended intubation. The intubation team, garbed in full Covid PPE augmented by our P100 masks, entered Kira's room and began setting up all our intubation equipment. I unlocked Kira's bed and pulled it away from the wall so that I could stand behind her to intubate. The head of the bed was up at 45 degrees, making it a little easier for her to breathe – my plan was to give her sedation medications and then drop the head of her bed flat for intubation just as she drifted off.

I was just finishing preparations at the head of the bed when Kira, facing away from me, raised her right hand like a schoolgirl with a question. For a moment, I didn't know what she was doing, but then she turned her head and looked back over her shoulder at me and I realized she wanted me to take her hand. I did and she gave me a squeeze. Through the hiss of the BiPAP mask, she shouted, "Thank you for praying with me." I was a bit surprised and touched, squeezed her hand back – *she had withdrawn a bit over the past 24 hours, perhaps putting all her effort into drawing each breath, but she was still 100% in there.* The intubation went without a hitch, but the fact that Kira required it meant her chances of surviving Covid had taken a serious hit. I mentally prepared for a long fight ahead.

Later that day, I walked by the room where George, the fitness nut, resided. It was dark, his computer shut down. He didn't look so chipper anymore. He was lying still in bed, locked in a grim battle to breathe behind his BiPAP mask – his O2 sat hovering in the high 80s, barely acceptable under the circumstances.

Prayer 39 (April 27, 2020)
Lord, thank you for giving us faith, by your grace, to get us through hard times.
When I'm in deep distress, I kneel before you and pray every day for deliverance. But when life goes well, I immediately begin to wander away.

Lord, please grant me true peace, that doesn't depend on my worldly circumstances. In good times or bad, Lord, help me hang on to this wisdom: I have no legitimate self-confidence except that which comes through your grace, your mercy, and your Holy Spirit.

Carlos kept me abreast of what seemed at the time like amazing events as Covid overran the Chicago suburban ICU where he worked. So far, things weren't nearly so bad in Arizona. I thought maybe our warm weather was protecting us – *a theory manifestly disproven a few months later when we became the global hotspot for Covid.*

I hoped we would straighten out our inadequate Covid testing capacity before our Covid caseload skyrocketed. The administration was trying to compensate for the huge shortfall of testing kits by rigidly controlling the process of ordering one. Physicians couldn't request a Covid test without first ordering a respiratory infection panel to rule out other (increasingly unlikely) conventional pathogens. If the panel came back negative, we could *request* administrative approval to order a Covid nasopharyngeal swab – *which some of you may now remember as the "nasal brain biopsy."* But this **test** was insensitive and there was a thirty percent chance that a patient infected with Covid would have a false negative nasal swab result, so a confirmatory Covid sputum "PCR" test (which detects viral genetic material) was required to be sure a pneumonia patient was truly negative for Covid. This test was sent out to a regional laboratory with a turnaround time of 5-7 days. The entire process translated to over a week of isolation procedures awaiting test results to rule out each patient suspected of having Covid.

A lot of patients were suspicious of having Covid that spring. Eighty-six-year-old Gale was admitted from a nursing home for treatment of atrial fibrillation (a rapid, irregular heart rhythm). Gale became short of breath and her O2 sat fell into the 80% range (dangerously low) during an attempted cardiac procedure to treat her atrial fibrillation. The procedure was aborted and Gale was transferred to the ICU. Although she didn't have a fever, her other findings were consistent with Covid. Residence in a nursing home was recognized as a strong risk factor for Covid. The dozens of healthcare workers who had encountered Gale so far this admission, including the staff of the ER and cardiac catheterization lab, as well as the transport team and admitting ICU nurses, had all been exposed to Gale wearing only surgical face masks.

I put on full Covid PPE, including my P100, before entering her room, and advised the nurses to do the same. Gale was lethargic, responding only briefly to painful nailbed pressure. Her lungs "sounded like a washing machine" through my stethoscope; they were so full of secretions. I decided to intubate her immediately.

Later that night, Gale spiked a fever to 101.3° and a chest X-ray showed pneumonia, further raising my suspicion she might have Covid. We transferred Gale to the Covid cohort zone in full isolation and requested administrative approval for a Covid test. Her nasopharyngeal swab came back negative 48 hours later, and her sputum Covid PCR test came back negative six days later. I was happy for Gale and for the staff who took care of her before she was put in isolation, but it was a costly and time-consuming process. Gale went on to recover over a few days and was discharged without a clear microbiological diagnosis.

Prayer 40 (April 28, 2020)
Father and Son, seated together in Heaven, we praise your holy names!
If only Earth could be like Heaven. But until we can be with you, we live in faith that by your will and sacrifice, you have prepared a place for us at your table.
Help us forgive each other as you first forgave us.
Help us resist earthly temptation; defend us from the evil one.
Let our daily lives glorify you.

[Another version of the Lord's Prayer]

I am grateful to have been raised in the Catholic church. I was an altar boy back in the early '70s and memorized *the Lord's Prayer* by fulsome repetition. I can still recite it without any thought whatsoever. But Jesus specifically instructed us *not* to pray by rote. The Lord's Prayer was worded perfectly by Jesus, yet re-wording it myself, even clumsily, helped me mentally process what it means.

Prayer 41 (April 29, 2020)
Holy Spirit, we need you more than ever.
When I am afraid, I put my trust in you. For you have told us: "I am the Lord your God, who takes hold of your right hand. Do not fear."
I worship you with reverence Lord, and rejoice with trembling.
I pay homage to the Son.
How blessed are we who take refuge in him!
[Taken from Psalm 56]

I was auscultating the heart of a woman with Covid pneumonia. My stethoscope tubing is 18 inches long, so that's how far away my eyes, nose and mouth were from her mouth when she suddenly coughed into my face. It happened so fast, she didn't have a chance to cover her mouth and I didn't have a chance to turn away. The plexiglass face shield of my P100 mask was splattered with her sputum and I briefly left the room, barely able to see through the faceplate, to carefully sterilize it with an antiviral solution. She later apologized more than necessary; that's what the mask was for.

A P100 had to be disinfected each time you took it off, so it was best to just leave it on as long as you could stand it. But even after we became accustomed to them, you could only wear a P100 for about an hour or two before you *had* to take it off; feel the cool room air on your face, maybe scratch your itchy chin. The surgical masks we wore outside the Covid cohort zone were much more comfortable – *I often forgot I had one on* – but far less protective.

But as the community attack rate of Covid rose, and hospital outbreaks were increasingly reported, contact with *any* person in the hospital became a potential threat. I began thinking I was more likely to catch Covid *outside* the Covid unit when my guard was down. So my partners and I began wearing N95 masks for all "non-Covid" patient care encounters. These N95s were meant to be disposable, but we were so short-supplied that the hospital started collecting used N95s, decontaminating them, and returning them to their previous owners for reuse. I never turned my daily N95 in, but hung it in my locker between uses, careful not to touch the contaminated outer surface of the mask while donning or duffing it.

Prayer 42 (April 30, 2020)
"Naked I came into this world and naked will I depart. The Lord gives and the Lord takes away. Blessed be the name of the Lord."

Job said it right. I was reminded of this when I took care of my Mom's last belongings: purse, keys, etc. – I was struck that she didn't need them anymore.

[This prayer from Job 1:21-22 and the brief subsequent commentary was offered by Peter M. on the anniversary of his mother's death – God rest her soul]

Prayer 43 (May 1, 2020)
Lord, creator of Heaven and Earth, King above all kings, we praise your holy name.
We pray that you will deliver us from this plague, that you will heal your people from this disease. We pray for our brothers and sisters in darkness.
Use us to help lead them into the light, so that they would return to you in worship. In Jesus' name.

This was the day that warplanes from Luke Air Force Base did a fly-over of Valley hospitals as a salute to frontline healthcare workers. I went out on the grass lawn in front of our hospital with a crowd of nurses, RTs and other hospital workers. Isaiah and Lynn called me over to hang with them, and I got my shoes wet because they were standing in a shallow puddle of sprinkler water on the lawn. The planes roared right over our heads, shaking the Earth. They were led by a huge KC-135 refueling tanker – then about 15 jet fighters followed in several small formations. There were F-16 Strike Eagles (still my favorite), F-35 Lightnings and possibly a few F-22 Raptors (although it was hard for me to keep those last two straight). They flew low, slow and LOUD. It's going to sound stupid, and it surprised me, but I have to admit I started to cry a little. Something about seeing those mighty warplanes was incredibly emotional; they were majestic and powerful and somehow stood for all that's good and strong in our country. If those planes were sent on a mission to fight evil, they would be the closest earthly thing to avenging angels, I can imagine.

Prayer 44 (May 2, 2020)
Almighty God, I thank you for the job you made for me to do today. May I find contentment in difficult work, whether it succeeds or fails here on Earth.
Grant that I would always look away from myself and towards the needs of my brothers.
Give me a servant's heart, like yours Jesus, so I can stand and bear the burden of the day like you did, full of thanks and praise to God for letting me join in his work!

George the jogger was sedated and on a ventilator today; his sharp mind and fighting attitude didn't count for anything anymore.

The insidious natural course of severe Covid pneumonia was becoming apparent. Kira continued to decline with each passing day. This was unexpected. Before Covid, reasonably-healthy patients like Kira with severe pneumonia caused by common pathogens (e.g., influenza virus or *Streptococcus pneumonia* bacteria) generally stabilized or recovered over a week or so on the ventilator. We were witnessing a much more relentless process with Covid pneumonia – patients continuing to worsen despite weeks on life support, their immune response impotent, possibly even *worsening* the damage caused by the virus. We didn't know it yet, but Kira's progressive downhill course was the rule than the exception with severe Covid.

Prayer 45 (May 3, 2020)
Thank you, Lord, for the Holy Spirit dwelling within us.
Show us more of your truth.
Thank you, Lord, for the beautiful world you made for our home: the wondrous Heavens and microscopic world, filled with mysteries for us to discover.
Thank you Lord for each other – you gave us each other to love – our friends, family, and everyone we meet or think of.
Thank you Lord for choosing us to be your children, for no other reason than because of your merciful grace.
Thank you for the faith to know that every day of my life is covered by the protection and provision of your love.

On this discouraging day, we could no longer maintain Kira's O2 sat despite the highest ventilator settings, and she passed away from progressive hypoxemia (low blood oxygen levels). On some internal emotional level, I didn't fully accept it. I had seen many hundreds of patients die throughout my career. And I knew Covid pneumonia was potentially fatal, but it just *didn't seem possible* that someone like Kira could die like this, right in front of our eyes. Despite our considerable technology, there was nothing we could do to stop it. It struck me that when Kira turned to me just prior to her intubation, took my hand and thanked me for praying with her; she uttered her last spoken words on this Earth.

Prayer 46 (May 4, 2020)
Let the book of your law be written upon my heart and let my mouth not depart from it.
Let my mind meditate upon, and my body obey your law, day and

night.
Make my way prosperous in accordance with your command.
Grant me strength and courage in the sure knowledge that the Lord
my God is with me wherever I go. [Joshua 1:8-9]

Prayer 47 (May 5, 2020)
How lovely is your dwelling place O Lord.
My soul yearns for the courts of the Lord.
Better is one day in your courts than a thousand elsewhere.
Even the sparrow has found a home - a place near your altar.
Blessed are those who dwell in your house; they are ever praising
you.
Blessed are those whose strength is in you, whose hearts are set on
pilgrimage. They go from strength to strength until each appears
before God.
[Psalm 84 abbreviated]

Although the Covid surge in Arizona was just beginning, it was already reaching proportions rarely before seen. On this day, six of the patients in our ICU had confirmed Covid pneumonia. This approximated the peak census of H1N1 influenza patients in our ICU during the "Swine flu" pandemic of 2009 – the worst previous adult pneumonia outbreak in the course of my career.

A report from Massachusetts General Hospital published on this date showed healthcare workers were twelve times more likely to catch Covid than the general population. Mayfield and I talked about it and decided we would take turns, week by week, one or the other of us taking *all* the Covid patients each day so that the other could periodically enjoy reduced exposure risk. No sense in both of us being exposed every day. This system was short-lived, as the surge worsened and Covid patients took up more and more of our effort – we would soon *both* be doing nothing but seeing Covid patients all day long.

Prayer 48 (May 6, 2020)
Now may the God of peace, the Great Shepherd who saved us

through the blood of his Son, our Lord Jesus Christ, equip us with everything good for doing his will, and work in us what is pleasing to him, for his glory, forever!

McKale was discharged to a rehabilitation facility, still a little groggy and emaciated but slowly progressing with physical therapy. A general axiom in the ICU is that a patient might require a week of rehabilitation for every day they spend on life support. If so, McKale, who had been in the ICU for 26 days, still had a long road ahead.

Prayer 49 (May 7, 2020)
Heavenly Lord, I pray that you will bless me this day.
Keep me healthy so that I can minister to the sick.
Show me the right way, so I can help guide the lost.
Strengthen my faith so that I can encourage those in despair.
Grant me a merciful heart so that I can forgive those who have done me wrong. And help me love my brothers and sisters through your Holy Spirit in me!

George passed away from Covid pneumonia; his jogging days were over.

Prayer 50 (May 8, 2020)
Dear Lord, you have brought us through 50 days of prayer, and our goal is 100. Turn these 100 days of prayer into thousands.
Let your Holy Spirit enlighten us every day, to look to you, our heavenly Father, for grace today and each day to come.
Sovereign King, holy is your name.
Let your kingdom come, and your will be done on Earth as it is in Heaven.
Give us this day our daily bread. We ask for just enough for today because we know you will always be there to provide for us again tomorrow.
We thank you forever for the sustenance and the salvation of our souls. We pray in Jesus's name.
[Another version of the Lord's Prayer]

Prayer 51 (May 9, 2020)

Dear Lord, my soul thirsts for you and my flesh faints for you, as in a dry and weary land where there is no water.

I remember you upon my bed and meditate on you in the watches of the night. So I have looked upon you in the sanctuary, beholding your power and glory.

Because your steadfast love is better than life, my lips will praise you. So I will bless you as long as I live, in your name I will lift up my hands.

I will praise you with joyful lips when I remember you in the morning and in the evening. For you have been my help and in the shadow of your wings, I will sing for joy.

My soul clings to you; your right hand upholds me.

I praise you, Lord Jesus.

[Psalm 63:1-8 abbreviated and updated]

I got a page from our transfer service about a 48-year-old Navajo man being seen in White River ER for Covid pneumonia, who needed a transfer for life support. I asked the ER doc why Covid was hitting the Indian nations so hard; he said this particular patient lived with eleven other people in a three-bedroom house.

I practiced my entire career in Arizona, taking care of many Native Americans along the way, and I have high regard for their strong sense of family, honest expression of sincere emotion, and strong faith in more than what meets the eye – whether through traditional religion or Christianity. They are some of the greatest people I was ever blessed to work for. But now we were seeing a heartbreaking over-representation of all Native American people in our ICU due to Covid. The Navajo Nation was especially hard-hit. I did some rough math and found that during the spring of 2020, Navajo Americans were at least twice as likely to get Covid and 3.5 times more likely to die from it compared to other Arizonans. But I had a hard time believing these statistics; it seemed much worse than that from our vantage point. I suspect cases in the Indian Nations may have been undercounted. Our hospital was located in a community where Covid was relatively uncommon so far. This allowed us to take care of large numbers of Native Americans transferred from Northern Arizona, where regional healthcare capacity had been overrun. By June, our hospital had taken more Covid transfers than any other in the state, and we were taking care of Covid patients from the Navajo, Apache, Pima, Yavapai, Maricopa, and Hopi nations.

Prayer 52 (May 10, 2020)
Lord, we ask you to fill us with compassion, kindness, humility, meekness and patience.
Help us bear with one another, and to forgive each other as you forgave us.
Fill our hearts with love, which binds everything together in perfect harmony, and let your peace rule in our hearts.
Let your word dwell in us richly, teaching and admonishing us in all wisdom.
And whatever we do, Lord, in word or deed, let it be in the name of the Lord Jesus, giving thanks to God the Father through him.
[Colossians 3:12-17 abbreviated]

Prayer 53 (May 11, 2020)
Almighty God, through your Holy Spirit, you have made me one with your saints in Heaven and on Earth – my Bible study brothers. Grant, in my time left on Earth, I may always be supported by this fellowship of love and prayer and be surrounded by their witness to your power and mercy.
I ask this in the name of Jesus, who made me worthy to ask it, and who lives and reigns forever.

Our Bible study, with a life span of over 25 years, thrived via Zoom during the pandemic for spiritual and *technological* reasons (all things working together for the Lord's plan). Although some of us older guys had trouble remembering to mute Zoom when they weren't speaking, sometimes with embarrassing/humorous results during bathroom breaks.

Prayer 54 (May 12, 2020)

Heavenly Father, when I think of the wonder of your great plan for our salvation, I fall on my knees before you – who has named every name in Heaven and on Earth – praying that out of the richness of your loving-kindness, you will strengthen me in my inner being with your spirit, so that Christ may dwell in my heart through faith.

And I pray that I may be rooted in love, that I might have strength to comprehend the breadth and length and height and depth of the love of Christ Jesus, love that surpasses knowledge, and be filled with the fullness that only you can give.

In the name of Christ I pray. [From Ephesians 3:14-20]

Not everyone we see in the unit is deathly ill. Most patients with strokes are admitted for at least 24 hours of observation, regardless of whether the stroke is severe. Even a small stroke can lead to life-threatening complications, which can be carefully monitored in the ICU. But sometimes, the least sick ICU patients can take up a lot of time.

Mr. Zeitmann was a 77-year-old man admitted for a small stroke, the location of which didn't affect speech, motor, or cognitive abilities but interfered with the flow of cerebral spinal fluid (CSF) that cushions the brain, thereby requiring an external CSF drain. This was considered a minor procedure for our neurosurgeons. I was warned by nurse Samantha that Zeitmann was a bit of a talker, but I thought it would be a nice change of pace since few of our ICU patients could get out more than a word or two.

"How are you doing, Mr. Zeitmann?"

"Well, I'm here in this hospital bed – in the ICU – so I guess not too good! Frankly, doctor, I'm a mess. See these legs?" he said, lifting one then the other in the air (there was nothing visibly wrong with his legs), "they were swollen like tree trunks last week. I saw my doctor and he told me to put my feet up. Four years of medical school and that's the advice he gives me! So at home, I have one of those, what do you call them? – ottomans. Yes, ottomans. So I put my feet up while I watch TV. And look! They're better, but now apparently, I have to use an ottoman every time I want to watch TV! – which isn't easily said as done in my house because we have two TVs but only one ottoman."

I interrupted, trying to ascertain whether the stroke had affected his ability to swallow, "Are you able to eat, OK?"

"Eat? Sure! I'd *like* to eat. But you should have seen what they gave me for breakfast! Cold toast! The butter wouldn't melt! Who can eat toast without butter? Cold coffee! I don't know why, with all the MRI scanners and everything they have around here why they can't figure out how to serve the coffee hot. Doctor, do you like cold coffee? – *feigning sincerity as though I really might like cold coffee.*

"Mr. Zeitmann, next time, just ask the nurse to microwave your coffee and food for you."

"What? And wait forever for them to come? I might starve to death waiting! I press this little button here, and nobody comes! Where is it?" He started rummaging about his twisted bedsheets, trying to find the nurse call button without success.

"Mr. Zeitmann, we can look for it later."

"Yes – you were asking about my breakfast; well, the toast was *burnt* too. I should have kept it to show to you. It was terrible, so I threw it out. It might still be in the garbage there somewhere if you don't believe me." He peered from bedside to bedside, trying to find the garbage can.

"It's OK, Mr. Zeitmann; I don't need to see the toast – I believe you. Are you having any pain?"

"Yes! Finally, someone asks! My real problem is my neck! My neck is hurting me terribly this morning." He grabbed the back of his neck to show me: "Here, right back here, terrible pain." *Now this was potentially important – neck pain could signal an infection of the CSF drain.*

"When did the neck pain start?"

"1983. We were driving across the country for our summer vacation. We drove to Oxnard, California, from St. Louis, Missouri. Do you know how far Oxnard is from St Louis? One thousand eight hundred and eighty-two miles!"

As the minutiae of this road trip were excruciatingly detailed, I became increasingly preoccupied with how much work I still had to do before the end of my shift. Somehow I had to extricate myself from the room without being rude. I tried the gambit of putting my stethoscope in my ears, indicating I wanted to listen to his heart. Maybe he would take the hint. Zeitmann stopped talking for just a second as I placed the stethoscope on his chest, but he was only catching his breath. He went right ahead talking. I couldn't understand him *or* hear his heart sounds. "Mr. Zeitmann, please hold on just a second while I listen. . ."

"Oh! OK – sorry, doctor," looking contrite.

I lifted the stethoscope off his chest and Zeitmann immediately resumed: "Anyway, I was telling you about these doctors in Oxnard, in the emergency room. They looked at my neck and did X-rays. Told me my neck was OK, but here I am, almost forty years later and it still hurts!"

I tried my second technique. I started backing away slowly towards the door while maintaining eye contact and nodding my head sympathetically. "I'm sorry about your neck."

"And the nurse! I asked her for something for the neck pain and she told me I could have a Tylenol – a Tylenol! Here I am in the hospital, in the ICU, and all they can give me is a Tylenol!"

I took another step back towards the door. "What do you take at home for your neck pain?" – *trying to figure out what previously worked for him so that I could perhaps prescribe it.*

"Nothing. I put up with it. You know why? Pills. You start taking pills, and you'll never stop. That's the problem with this whole world; there's a pill for everything."

Although I hadn't been able to ask all the questions I would like, I had been observing Zeitmann closely, noting the movements of his eyes, facial muscles, arms and legs and the cadence of his speech. He was basically doing OK neurologically. I took another step back towards the door and freedom. He was still talking; he would *keep* talking until long after I had left the room and started down the hall.

Prayer 55 (May 13, 2020)
Lord, you have been our dwelling place throughout all generations. Before the mountains were born, or you brought forth the Earth, from everlasting to everlasting, you are God.
You turn men back to dust, saying "Return to dust O sons of men."
For 1000 years in your sight is like a day that has just gone by, or like a watch in the night.
You have set our iniquities before you, our secret sins in the light of your presence. Who knows the power of your anger? For your wrath is great as the fear that is due you.
Teach us to number our days rightly, so that we may gain a heart of wisdom.
Relent O Lord, have compassion on your servants.
Satisfy us in the morning with your unfailing love so that we may sing for joy – make your deeds be shown to your servants, your splendor to your children, and may the favor of the Lord rest upon us.
[Psalm 90 abbreviated]

Prayer 56 (May 14, 2020)
O God, Eternal King, who divides the day from the darkness, and has turned the shadow of death into the light of morning: I pray that this day you incline my heart to keep your commandments, driving temptation from my mind.
Guide my feet in the path of peace, that having done your will with cheerfulness while it was day, I can give you thanks when the night comes, for living in your presence through Jesus Christ our Lord.

Our ICU census was 22, eight with Covid pneumonia. I had never seen eight ICU patients with the same infectious disease at the same time before, not even during the 2009 Swine flu pandemic.

Prayer 57 (May 15, 2020)
Lord, so many are suffering now and worried about the future.
But your servant spirit is with us.
A nurse reminded me today how you came into our world. Not worried about her own safety, she bravely came to serve.
Thank you, Lord, for sending your spirit of loving-kindness down to us in our hour of need.

By mid-May, we were running a daily census of over ten Covid pneumonia patients on life support – about half of our ICU service. One of the infection control principles we adopted was to enter Covid rooms as seldom as possible. IV pumps and ventilator control circuits were wired up *outside* the patient's rooms. All procedures were performed with minimal staff. Nurses were carrying-out tasks such as food delivery to prevent food service workers from risking exposure. So I was shocked this day to find nurse Lynn lingering in the room of a 60-year-old Covid patient named Lily, simply to wash her hair.

Lily had beautiful long salt-and-pepper colored hair, which Lynn was brushing, fanned out across the pillow to dry. Meanwhile, they were chatting together like old high school friends. For a moment, it just looked like two girls playing hair-dresser together. It was such an unexpected and kind act, so far removed from my state of anxiety that I started crying a little. I told Lynn later; I couldn't decide if this was one of the dumbest or sweetest things I had ever seen, *although it was obviously the latter.*

A few days later, Lily took a turn for the worse and had to be intubated. A week later, she experienced severe barotrauma (her lungs began to rupture from the pressure the ventilator was exerting on them). A week after that, Lily was in a proning bed, on 100% oxygen. She passed away shortly thereafter. As is often the case with the small kindnesses of our ICU nurses, having her hair washed by Lynn might have been the last act of human kindness Lily experienced in this life.

May 15, 2020. *Lynn washing Lily's hair as seen through the closed glass door of the Covid isolation room*

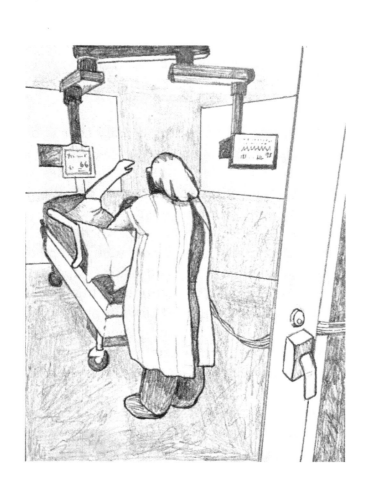

Prayer 58 (May 16, 2020)
Praise the Lord my soul, who forgives all our sins, who redeems our life from the pit, who satisfies all our desires with good things.
The Lord is compassionate, slow to anger, and abounding in love.
He does not treat us as our sins deserve or repay us according to our iniquities, for as high as the Heavens are above the Earth, so great is his love for those who fear him.

As far as the East is from the West, so far has he removed our transgressions from us.
The Lord has established his throne in Heaven in his kingdom rules over all. Praise the Lord my soul!
[Paraphrase of Psalm 103]

Prayer 59 (May 17, 2020)
When the Lord restored the fortunes of his people, it was like we were in a dream. Our mouths were full of laughter, our tongues with shouts of joy.
The Lord has done great things for us, let us be glad!
Restore our fortunes O Lord, like streams in the desert.
Those who sow in tears will reap with shouts of joy.
[From Psalm 126]

Prayer 60 (May 18, 2020)
God protect and bless the Navajo, Hopi, Pima, and all the Indian nations, with whom we share this beautiful state of Arizona that you created. Deliver them from Covid.
Bless their families, bless their homes, bless their land, and all they hold dear.
Bless their spirits – give them even more strength, resilience, hope and faith.
Let your Holy Spirit abide in all their nations.
Shower down the humility, forgiveness and loving-kindness of our Lord Jesus upon all your children in Arizona, native and immigrant.
Let us accept the truth in our hearts that we are all brethren, your children on Earth.
Forgive us for our transgressions. Grant us unity and love.

Today I took care of an elderly Apache man *and* his adult grandson, both on ventilators in adjacent ICU rooms. The elder would not survive his ICU stay.

It was also the day I admitted one of the youngest patients we saw die from Covid. He was a stubborn 27-year-old Navajo man named Anderson, with no significant past medical history. Anderson and his wife had come down with fever, cough and anosmia (loss of sense of smell) about a week earlier. He was seen in a rural ER where a rapid Covid test was positive and his O2 sat was 80%. They urged admission, but Anderson left "AMA" (against medical advice). Within 24 hours, he could barely breathe, finally gave in and called 911. His O2 sat had fallen into the 70% range!

Although he was having shaking chills, and in obvious respiratory distress with blue lips, Anderson was still pretty stubborn when he arrived in our ICU. He refused to wear a BiPAP mask, didn't want me to put the lights on to examine him, and wouldn't consent to treatment with convalescent plasma. Sam had to repeatedly re-enter his room to replace the BiPAP mask, which he kept taking off, exposing herself to his coughing fits each time. Within an hour of his arrival, it was clear he wouldn't survive the night without intubation.

Sam asked me to consent Anderson for intubation – a standard practice in which we explain the risks/benefits of the procedure and request permission to proceed with respect to the patient's autonomy. I hesitated. *Anderson was 27. He needed life support. What if he refused? I was tired of arguing with him, and I wasn't going to let him die before we had a chance to see how he might respond. I decided to do something I had never even considered before.*

"I'm not going to consent him, Sam. He might say no. We're not going to just stand by and watch him die. We are going to sedate him and intubate him." I looked her right in the eye, inviting objection. I purposely didn't explicitly ask for Sam's approval – *let this decision be on me.* But I knew Sam would not have gone along with me if she didn't agree.

Prayer 61 (May 19, 2020)
No matter what each day brings, Lord, you give us what we need to prevail thru your Holy Spirit in us.
All things on Heaven and Earth work together to achieve your ends. All knees shall bend, the willing and the unwilling.

Yet you listen to our prayers. Please use us as you see fit.
We trust your loving-kindness and mercy. Your will be done.

When I examined Anderson first thing the next morning, I heard and felt crepitus in his neck (crackling of gas bubbles under his skin that reminded me of Rice Krispies in milk) – a sign that his lungs were starting to rupture after just 12 hours on the vent! (This became a recurrent Catch-22 in the ventilator management of Covid pneumonia patients – their stiff lungs required high pressure to inflate, but the high pressure further injured their lungs). To make matters worse, Anderson's morning labs indicated kidney failure – worsening so rapidly that I wasn't sure I believed it until I had his blood redrawn, confirming the results.

It was clear that Anderson would not survive without the highest level of life support available: ECMO (extracorporeal membrane oxygenation) – a machine that completely takes the place of the lungs, injecting oxygen directly into the heart through IV lines as big around as your finger. ECMO is only provided by a small number of hospitals with the highest level of specialization. Our hospital wasn't one of these. If Anderson was going to get ECMO, we would have to get him stable enough to survive an ambulance transport to an ECMO center about ten minutes away.

We began to make arrangements and with that cooking, I ran around to see as many of my other patients as I could. But around noon, the code bells went off, and I recognized the location announced by the overhead emergency intercom with dread – room 352: *Anderson's room!*

The code team, which I was leading that day, was backed-up outside the door donning P100 masks, gowns and gloves and piling into the room as fast as possible. Anderson had gone into a heart rhythm called pulseless electrical activity (PEA) – in which the heart has an electrical rhythm on the monitor but is not *physically* pumping any blood. CPR was already underway when I entered the room. I strongly suspected one of Anderson's lungs had completely ruptured, and called for the ultrasound machine, as we pushed intravenous epinephrine and continued CPR without obvious benefit.

Every two minutes during a code, CPR is interrupted for 5-10 seconds to perform a rhythm check and switch out the person performing CPR – *it's harder than you think to do good CPR for 2 minutes, especially in a P100 mask and a plastic gown.* It was during one of these brief pauses that I was able to determine with our ultrasound machine that neither of Anderson's lungs had ruptured. As I worked through the list of other possible causes of code arrest, the answer was handed to me by June, the RT on service who had sent off a blood gas analysis on her own initiative about ten minutes earlier. Anderson's blood was incredibly acidotic at pH 6.8 – caused by the combination of his lung's inability to exhale carbon dioxide and his failing kidneys. *No wonder he crashed. I should have anticipated this.*

We gave bicarbonate intravenously to temporarily neutralize the acidosis and turned the ventilator up to the highest settings we dared to clear carbon dioxide. Fifteen minutes into the code, Anderson regained an erratic rapid heart rhythm (atrial fibrillation), pushing a faint pulse – "return of spontaneous circulation" was achieved, but his blood pressure was dangerously low. I shocked him into a more stable sinus rhythm just as the ECMO transport team arrived. They nearly turned right around and left when they saw what was going on. We begged them to stay with us as long as they could, in the hope we could stabilize Anderson adequately to survive transport. ECMO was surely his only chance now.

Samantha and the transport team worked feverishly over the next hour to make that happen. Finally, Anderson's blood pressure and oxygen saturation were "good enough" under the circumstances to attempt the transfer. Grant, a Family Practice resident, who had been expressly forbidden from seeing Covid patients under the policy of his training program, volunteered to suit-up in full PPE and travel in the ambulance with

Anderson, carrying a bag of ACLS drugs in case Anderson coded again. Grant got a chance to direct another round of ACLS when Anderson briefly lost his pulse just upon arrival at his destination. Anderson was successfully put on full ECMO life support about an hour later.

May 19^{th,} 2020. *Nurse Samantha raised her right arm in victory after providing ACLS and shocking Anderson. He was now stable enough to be transferred for ECMO. The transport team is in the room celebrating with her.*

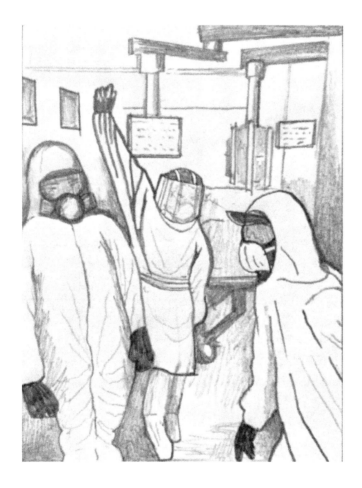

One of our family practice residents, Grant, dressed up in PPE to accompany Anderson in the transport ambulance.

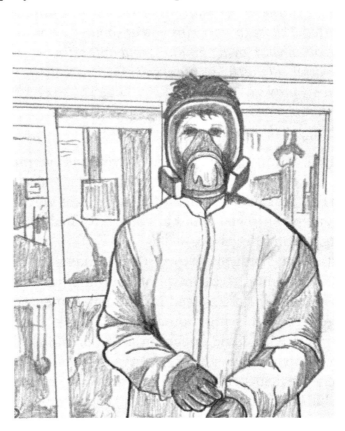

Prayer 62 (May 20, 2020)
I sought the Lord, and he answered me, and delivered me from all my fears.
The eyes of the Lord are toward the righteous and his ears toward their cry.
Many are the afflictions of the righteous, but the Lord delivers him out of them all.
The Lord redeems the life of his servants; none who take refuge in him will be condemned.
[From Psalm 34].

Prayer 63 (May 21, 2020)
*I lay awake in the lonely watches of the night. Stiff-necked and
cold-hearted, I chose to worry instead of coming to you.*
I had forgotten your loving-kindness and authority.
*I had forgotten all the times before you saved me – all the times you
answered my prayers.*
But then, I remembered – the Lord is my shepherd.
Once again, you lifted me up!

Today I admitted Clarice, a 93-year-old woman with
Alzheimer's dementia and Covid pneumonia. I also met her
son Marty. You can't be much of a healthcare worker if you
can't get along with just about anyone, but I had trouble with
Marty right from the get-go.

A little past medical history: Clarice had spent most of
the past four months in hospitals or nursing homes. She
was most recently hospitalized for influenza pneumonia and
discharged to a nursing home for only five days before
coming down with Covid pneumonia. She previously suffered
a stroke which affected her ability to swallow and had
a severely weakened heart due to coronary artery disease,
chronic kidney disease, colitis, chronic back pain from spinal
stenosis, malnourishment and (unsurprisingly) depression.
She weighed 84 pounds. I was grateful that she had previously
requested do-not-resuscitate status (DNR) because I dreaded
the thought of intubating her or, worse – *actually coding her*,
which would likely break every one of her fragile ribs.

Over the past several days, Clarice's Covid pneumonia
worsened, and she went into septic shock from secondary
bacterial pneumonia* requiring "pressors" (drugs that keep the
blood pressure from getting too low). The bacterial infection
set up shop in the pleural space around her right lung,
filling it with pus and requiring a chest tube for drainage.
Placement of a chest tube was a painful procedure that we had
misgivings about performing on a frail 93-year-old woman.

Clarice required BiPAP and became increasingly withdrawn and uncommunicative as her chances of survival dwindled. But she tried to make her wishes known. She weakly fought the nurses during any procedure: suctioning of her throat, placement of an IV, a urinary catheter. The nurses heard her saying, "I'm done. I'm done," repeatedly through the BiPAP mask. But Clarice wasn't coherent anymore and future decision-making legally passed to her closest relative – her son Marty.

I called him to explain the situation but couldn't get far before Marty cut me off. He had access to his mom's EMR (electronic medical record) and he seemed more interested in impressing me with how much he knew rather than hearing what I had to say. He rattled off her lab values from that morning and wanted to know what my plan was for each abnormality, even those that were inconsequential. I thought he was pretty well-informed about the trees but didn't understand the forest at all. After silently listening to his report to me on how his mother was doing, I gave up trying to inform him and redirected the discussion toward the issue of his mother's DNR, which I wanted to be sure he was aware of.

"Oh, that? – I am my mother's medical power of attorney. Now that she can't speak for herself anymore, I'm rescinding the DNR. She wants everything done."

I was taken aback. "Hmmm, Marty – I have to say, that doesn't seem advisable given your mother's condition and her expressed prior wishes. You're supposed to represent *her* wishes, not your own."

"Well, she wasn't herself when she made that decision, and I know what's best for her. I also think she needs another one of those chest tubes on her other lung."

"Marty, that wouldn't make sense; your mom doesn't have a fluid accumulation to drain on that side. Putting a chest tube won't do anything but cause her pain."

I could tell he didn't like being corrected. I recommended comfort care – withdrawing life support and providing pain relief, allowing for a natural outcome. I did this more to carry out my duty to Clarice than with any hope Marty would agree, and of course, he didn't. It was with a heavy heart that I hung up the phone. I feared that the only thing we would henceforth accomplish was to prolong Clarice's suffering.

[*Secondary bacterial pneumonia is a common complication of severe viral pneumonia. It has been recognized for over a hundred years that some patients with influenza pneumonia start to recover, then suddenly decline due to bacterial superinfection of their lungs. The most common pathogen is Staphylococcus aureus, but a variety of other bacteria are also culprit. These bacteria are opportunists, taking advantage of the disarray of natural host defenses in the aftermath of viral pneumonia; thriving in the wreckage, these bacteria often finish the patient off. Turns out, Covid was just as inviting to bacterial superinfection as influenza, maybe even more so.]

Prayer 64 (May 22, 2020)
Lord, you sent from on high, and drew me out of many waters.
You rescued me from my strong enemy and from those who hated me, for they were too many for me. They confronted me on the day of my calamity, but you were my support.
You brought me out into a broad place and you rescued me because you delighted in me!
[From Psalm 18]

Prayer 65 (May 23, 2020)
Lord, when our Bible study started more than 25 years ago, your plans for it were so much greater than anything we could have imagined.
I don't have a brother in the flesh, but through your mercy and love, you have given me brothers in the Spirit.
Thanks to you, Father and Son. I want to cry when I consider your grace and kindness to me, a wretched man.
Strengthen and bless our brotherhood even more, Lord.

Bring us together so we can trust each other, encourage and advise each other in the Holy Spirit, pray together, and help each other when need arises – like true brothers.
How rich is our inheritance as your children on Earth!

When you get grey hair, you're entitled to certain workplace idiosyncrasies. Ever since the HIPAA (Health Information Portability and Accountability Act) law came into effect, hospital staff have been discouraged from using patients' names in clinical discourse. In almost all verbal interactions, staff in our hospital refer to patients by their room numbers rather than their names. To me, it didn't make any sense to "not to name names" when engaging in patient-care communication – it's potentially dangerous to obscure the patient's identity and it's dehumanizing.

"Room 362 is having some leg pain, doctor Eckshar. Can I get an order for pain meds?"

"What is the patient's name?" – *I made a point of asking, although I knew Ellen McDonnell was the patient in room 362.*

"Name? Oh, I don't . . . " looking discombobulated. "Oh, let's see . . . um, Mrs. McDonnell."

"*Ellen!* – yes, I'll order Ellen McDonnell some PRN pain meds."

I worried at times that I was being an obstinate jerk about this. But it was so ingrained in our culture to avoid referring to a patient by their name, I felt hardheadedness was called for on my part to combat it. I don't know if I made any lasting effect on the dehumanizing practice of identifying a person by their room number, but it wasn't for lack of trying.

Prayer 66 (May 24, 2020)
Heavenly Father, maker of Heaven and Earth, your word is law.
Let your plan unfold. Have mercy on us.
Send down a gentle rain to cool us and make the world green.
Give us a new clean heart – pleasing to your Holy Spirit.
Protect us from the consequences of our transgressions through your holy blood. Give us peace and don't let us fall.

We cannot stand without you.
Father, we call out to you in the name of your holy Son.
[Another version of the Lord's prayer]

I saw an 88 year old patient named Raymond with severe heart damage from coronary artery disease, and diffuse lung fibrosis (scarring) from radiation therapy he had received for cancer. Ray had a living will stipulating DNR status, but when he fell and broke his hip, his wife Pearl decided to rescind it temporarily, so that he could be intubated for hip surgery. Over the three days since his surgery, he went into heart failure and had been unable to come off the vent. Ray was frail and looked his age. He was completely deaf and kept his eyes closed at all times (in fact, when I tried to open his eyelids to examine them, he fought me – the only purposeful thing I could get him to do). He was requiring 50% oxygen and his chest X-ray showed severe infiltrates. He was already receiving empirical* antibiotics and steroids; I added a strong diuretic. [*"Empirical"* *in this context essentially means that we weren't sure exactly what we were treating with the antibiotics or steroids.*]

He was between a "rock and a hard place" – he had too much fluid on board for his heart and lungs to handle, but barely enough to keep his kidneys functioning. It didn't look very hopeful to me.

Ray's wife Pearl seemed like a very loving wife and good decision-maker; I liked her from the minute I met her. But she was dispirited and beginning to feel uneasy about rescinding the DNR. She seemed close to a decision to let him go. "I hope I did the right thing – letting them do surgery - Ray didn't want the ventilator, but he always bounced back before. I just hoped we could have a *little* more time together."

"I think you made a good decision Pearl, out of love. I promise we won't leave Ray in this predicament. What would you think of giving me 48 hours to get Ray in as good a shape as possible and then we honor his DNR and take him off the vent "sink or swim?" This will give him a fighting chance, but if he doesn't breathe on his own by then, we let nature take it's course. You can sit with him, and I promise I won't let him suffer." We agreed to this plan without much debate – seemingly on the same wavelength.

Prayer 67 (May 25, 2020)
I cry out to you, Lord, from the dark watches of the night, lost and surrounded by adversity. From your mighty throne in Heaven, you heard my cry.
You singled me out, in all the universe, and judged me worthy of the purpose for which you made me, and the blood of your Son.
You reached down from Heaven and put your hand on my head.
Of what can I be afraid?
You put my feet down on a straight and beautiful path.
I praise your holy name!

Ray looked about the same. The diuretic hadn't accomplished much, so I increased the dose. I touched base with Pearl again and confirmed our plan. She asked again if I thought we were doing the right thing, keeping Ray on the vent like this against his wishes, and I reassured her that I thought it was OK for just one more day. Ray was in no distress. Pearl related, "We've been married 65 years, and two of them were good, but not consecutively!" (laughing). "We've been blessed to have all this time together. We really have had a great life."

Unfortunately, I wasn't too hopeful about our upcoming extubation attempt, wishing Ray would show more spunk. Toward the end of my shift I went through his chart one last time and noticed that someone had started him on a nightly sleeping medication on admission. It was a pretty strong one for an 88 year old guy, so I discontinued it.

That night Jean prayed as she did every night: "*Lord bless Anthony, and bless all his patients and their families.*"

Prayer 68 (May 26, 2020)

Bless you, God and Father of our Lord Jesus Christ.
According to your great mercy, you allowed us to be born again, to a living hope through the resurrection of our Lord Jesus, from death to an inheritance that is imperishable.
By God's power we are being guarded through faith for a salvation ready to be revealed in the last time.
In this we rejoice, though now, for a while if necessary, we have been grieved by various trials, so that the tested genuineness of our faith may be found to result in praise, honor and glory at the revelation of Jesus Christ.
Though we do not see him, we love him. Though we do not see him, we believe in him and rejoice with joy that is inexpressible.
And filled with glory, obtaining the outcome of our faith: the salvation of our souls. [1 Peter 3-9]

When I got into work the next morning, Mayfield informed me that Ray had awoken at 1 am that morning and successfully self-extubated (pulled out his own ETT)! He was only requiring a small amount of oxygen. I stopped by his room and of course Pearl was sitting at his bedside holding his hand. She smiled, excited, "Ray woke up Dr. Eckshar – even gave me a little kiss! Go on, wake him up and see."

Ray looked asleep. I called out his name with no reaction, then remembered he was deaf. I laid my hand on his shoulder and his eye's popped open. They were brilliant blue and fixed mine with a piercing gaze. I held out my right hand; he grinned and shook it firmly, perhaps showing off just a little. His smile lit up the room and took 20 years off his visage.

Pearl asked, "What do you make of this?

"Well Pearl, I've heard it said, 'Man plans and God laughs'." She knew the expression and it made her smile again. I didn't know what the days ahead would bring for Ray and Pearl, but at least they had a *little more time together* as Pearl had wished-for, to hold hands and maybe share another kiss.

Prayer 69 (May 27, 2020)

Heavenly Father, your name is holy and your word is law in Heaven and on Earth.

Your Son, our Lord and Savior, Jesus Christ, told us 2000 years ago that your kingdom is at hand, and through your Holy Spirit, who has been gifted us through your grace, and who speaks through us and for us, we have become the holy soldiers of your kingdom on Earth – your advance guards in hostile territory.

Part of me is scared to say it, but, "Bring it on Lord". Let your kingdom come.

Provide our needs today Lord.

Our sins are washed away by Jesus's blood – how can we then fail to forgive each other?

Sanctify us Lord, and protect us from Satan.

All glory to you, in Heaven and on Earth, forever.

[Another version of the Lord's Prayer].

Prayer 70 (May 28, 2020)

Lord, hear my cry for mercy, come to my relief.

Do not bring your servant to judgment, for no one living is righteous before you without your Holy Spirit.

My spirit fails within me, my heart is dismayed – but then I remember the days long ago.

I meditate on all your works and consider what your hands have done and I spread out my hands to you.

My soul thirsts for you like a parched land.

Answer me quickly O Lord – do not hide your face from me.

In the morning, bring me word of your unfailing love, for I have put my trust in you.

Show me the way I should go, for to you I lift up my soul.

Rescue me O Lord, for I hide myself in you.

[Psalm 143 abbreviated]

I admitted Jameson, a 65-year-old man with metastatic lung cancer. Jameson previously failed all standard cancer treatments and was suffering unremitting pain from metastases in his spine and ribs. He had been diagnosed with brain mets six months previously, which initially responded to therapy. But a more recent brain CT demonstrated relapse of multiple enlarging tumors. As a result, Jameson declined into a confused delirium. You didn't have to be a doctor to know his life was over – he was cachectic, disheveled, mute, his thin face ceaselessly contorted in apparent pain. His limbs were wasted – I could almost encircle his entire calf in my grip. He had a tart smell to him. I've never come across this in any medical text, but had noticed this smell before in patients with life-threatening neurological diseases. The association might only have been my imagination, but I took this odor as another bad omen.

I talked with Isaiah about Jameson's pain med orders and we adjusted them as best we could to provide him comfort. Patients show wide variation in their response to narcotics, and it often takes some trial and error before getting the right dose – ameliorating pain without depressing breathing. ICU monitoring made this process safer. I left with this, "Isaiah, if Jameson needs more, give it – I'll sign for it." I trusted Isaiah and I didn't want Jameson suffering unnecessarily while we were trying to figure things out.

Then I checked Jameson's code status: *Full code.* No matter how long some patients have battled a terminal medical condition, many arrive in the ICU in their last few days without ever having had a conclusive discussion about code status. Full code status was assigned by default, meaning that when Jameson's heart stopped beating, I would be obliged to perform CPR and put him on life support, prolonging his death process and suffering even though his cancer was untreatable. I imagined how Jameson's ribs would feel breaking under the palms of my hands as I administered chest compressions. I had experienced that tactile sensation too many times in the past. I didn't ever want to ever again.

Jameson's next-of-kin was his 92-year-old mother. Here I came, a stranger calling to ask her permission to let her son die when his time came – what a disheartening proposition for the old gal. *No one should live so long as to see their children die.*

Her name, Amelia, and phone number were in our EMR. She picked up the landline number on the seventh ring – *I figured she might need a little extra time to get to her phone.*

"Amelia – Hi. My name is Dr. Eckshar – I'm one of the doctors taking care of your son Jameson at the hospital."

"OK, doctor?"

"Listen, Amelia, I'm really sorry to tell you this, but your son is doing badly. You know about cancer in his brain?"

"Yes."

"It looks like it has grown again. We don't have any more effective treatment for it. We're giving him pain medicine and steroids to reduce the swelling in his brain, but I think we are fighting a losing battle . . . It looks to me like he is near the end of his rope. It's a hard thing for me to ask you – but I *need* to ask you, Amelia, what would your son want us to do if he stops breathing, or his heart stops? . . . Would he want us to try CPR, to pump on his chest and put him on life support?" *What a cruel thing to ask – there was no proper choice of works to soften this contemplation of her son's death*

Amelia didn't answer at first, perhaps composing herself. "No. No life support. That would be selfish of me," her voice quavering. "I depend on Jameson – we take care of each other." She hesitated, "He's all I have left. He's talked before about taking his own life. He's suffered so much – the only reason he is going through treatment now is me. No. I couldn't do that to him, doctor."

"OK, Amelia. I'm so sorry to have to talk to you about such a difficult thing. I'm praying for you and your son. His nurse and I will make sure he isn't suffering."

"Thank you, doctor – and thanks for your prayers."

We changed our goal of Jameson's therapy from prolonging life to preventing suffering – a protocol we call "comfort care." Isaiah and I were at least able to ease the look of pain off Jameson's face before he passed away a day later. What a brave and selfless woman Amelia was.

Prayer 71 (May 29, 2020)
Jesus is patient. Jesus is kind.
When Jesus was human, he did not envy, nor was he prideful.
Jesus is never self-seeking but does all for the glory of his Father.
Jesus is not easily angered. He keeps no record of our wrongs.
He rejoices in the truth.
He always protects, always gives us another chance, and always perseveres. Jesus never fails.
One day, everything that passes as wisdom in our world will pass away, and only three things will remain: faith, hope and the love of Christ.
But the greatest of these is the love of Christ.
[From 1 Corinthians 13]

In stark contrast, Clarice, the 93-year-old woman with Alzheimer's dementia and Covid pneumonia, underwent tracheostomy (a surgical breathing tube placed into her trachea for long-term ventilator support) at the insistence of her son. Over the next week, a surgical feeding tube was placed through the wall of her stomach and she was transferred to a nursing home. We never heard from her or her son Marty again. But I remembered Clarice and prayed for peace for her.

SUMMER SURGE 2020: COMPASSION

Although summer wouldn't *officially* start for another 3 weeks, the high temperature reached 111 degrees and 700 people were hospitalized for Covid in Phoenix this week, for all practical purposes marking the beginning of the Summer Covid surge.

Prayer 72 (May 30, 2020)
Dear Lord, let us and all the Earth make a joyful noise to you.
Let us serve you with gladness. Dear Jesus, we come into your presence singing!
Help us to know that you Lord are God.
It is you who made us and we are your people – the sheep of your pasture.
Today Lord, we enter your gates with thanksgiving and your courts with praise. For you Lord are good and your steadfast love endures forever – your faithfulness extends to all generations.
[From Psalm 100]

For the first time, fully half of the patients in our ICU (12 of 24) were on life support because of Covid pneumonia, and I did nothing that day but see Covid patients for my entire 12-hour ICU shift.

One of our patients, Ethan, wasn't doing too bad so far. He required high-flow oxygen but was alert – able to eat and talk a little. I was curious and asked him how he caught Covid – a question I had begun asking all Covid patients well enough to talk. Many knew the circumstances. But Ethan said he didn't know. "How would anyone know that?"

I said, "Different ways – some had a family member who was ill, or maybe came in contact with someone coughing at work."

Ethan looked pensive. "Well, it was kind of weird the day I got sick. I went to work and I was the only one that showed up that day. Everyone else in the office had called in sick – *all seven of them.*"

"Do you guys wear masks in the office?"

"Well yes and no, we wore masks *to* the office, but once we got there, of course, we took them off."

Prayer 73 (May 31, 2020)
Heavenly father, we come before you in the spirit of supplication.
As sinners, we know we have much for which to repent, but as beloved children, we know we have great reason to hope in your abundant mercy.
As members of a society plagued by opposition to your gospel, we implore your help to work towards a society where discrimination, racism, hatred, division and rejection of your love are replaced by faith, hope and charity in the communion of all your saints, on Earth and in Heaven.
May your kingdom come Lord Jesus amen.
[Dr. Martin Luther King Jr.]

On this day, protests over the death of George Floyd escalated in 75 cities around the United States, including Minneapolis, New York, Los Angeles, Chicago and Washington DC, at the gates of the White House. Fiery clashes erupted between protestors and police. Thousands were arrested. Nineteen people died in the protests.

Prayer 74 (June 1, 2020)
Bless our God all you people.
Let the sound of his praise be heard in the land.
He who has kept our souls among the living will not let our feet slip. For you, O God, have tested us; you have tried us as silver is tempered in a furnace.
You laid a crushing burden on our backs. We went through fire and water, but you brought us out to a place of abundance.

[from Psalm 66]

Prayer 75 (June 2, 2020)
Heavenly Lord, you have brought me to the beginning of a new day.
As the world is renewed again, I ask you to renew my heart with your strength and purpose.
Forgive my errors of yesterday and guide me to walk closer in your footsteps.
This is the day I begin my life anew; shine through me so that every person I meet may feel your presence in my soul.
Take my hand, precious Lord, for I cannot make it by myself.
Through Christ, I pray and live.

Prayer 76 (June 3, 2020)
The Lord is gracious and compassionate, slow to anger and rich in love.
The Lord has compassion for all he has made.
All your works praise you, Lord.
Your faithful people praise you, so that all people may know of your mighty acts and the glorious splendor of your everlasting kingdom.
The Lord is trustworthy in all he promises and faithful in all he does.
The Lord upholds all who fall and lifts up all who are bowed down.
The Lord is near to all who call on him.
He fulfills the desires of those who fear him; he hears their cry and saves them.
The Lord watches over all who love him.
My mouth will speak in praise of the Lord.
Let every creature praise his holy name forever.
[Psalm 145 abbreviated]

One of our Covid pneumonia patients, Lambert, a 63-year-old Navajo man who became ill a week after taking his grandchildren on a fishing trip, had been slowly losing ground over the past two weeks. Lambert now needed the highest level of mechanical ventilation: 100% oxygen, at the highest pressure we dared to apply. We put him in a proning bed and his O2 sat begrudgingly rose to the mid 80% range – acceptable only given the dire circumstances.

Prayer 77 (June 4, 2020)
I will sing of the steadfast love of the Lord forever; I will make known his faithfulness to all generations.
Let the Heavens praise your wonders O Lord, your faithfulness in the assembly of the holy ones! For who in the skies can be compared to the Lord? Who among the heavenly beings is like the Lord?
O God, greatly to be feared and awesome above all around him.
You rule the raging sea, when its waves rise, you calm them!
Righteousness and justice are the foundations of your throne; steadfast love and faithfulness go before you.
[Psalm 89 abbreviated]

Lambert's kidneys failed, and we were forced to contemplate placing a large-bore dialysis IV (almost the thickness of a Bic ballpoint pen) in his neck. But the IV couldn't be inserted with Lambert proned. In order to get the line in, we would have to turn Lambert face-up.

On rounds that day, Lambert's nurse Lynn expressed her opinion that putting in the dialysis catheter might be too dangerous. I always listened carefully to the opinions of the nurses and the RTs but ultimately had to make my own decision. I reassured Lynn; we could supine Lambert and get the line in as fast as possible. It would probably be OK. We didn't have much of a choice anyway – Lambert would certainly die without dialysis. It took a while to prepare for the procedure, and the line team was still futzing-around, getting ready to supine Lambert when my shift ended and I headed home. Joyce was on call that night.

Prayer 78 (June 5, 2020)
Lord, the great and awesome God, who keeps his covenant with those who love him.
You are righteous, but this day our people, our leaders, and our

ancestors are covered with shame because we have sinned against you.
Disaster has come on us, yet we have not sought the favor of the Lord our God by turning from our sins and attending to your truth.
But in keeping with all your boundless mercy, turn away your wrath from your people.
Now, our God, hear the prayers of your servants. For your sake, Lord, look with favor on us.
We do not beseech you because we are deserving, but because of the blood of your Son.
Lord listen! Lord forgive! Lord, hear and act!
For your sake, my God, do not delay, because your people bear your name. [A further adaptation of Daniel's prayer. Daniel 9]

First thing when I arrived at the hospital the next morning, I bumped into a night shift ICU nurse in the hallway and learned that Lambert coded and died when he was supined for his dialysis line, as Lynn predicted he might. He received ACLS for about 25 minutes before the code was called (efforts to revive him ceased).

I had never before seen a patient die from merely changing their position in bed. My decision to override Lynn's concern had been completely and fatally off-base. I was humbled by the lethality of Covid pneumonia and the limitations of my foresight. As doctors, we were trained to make life-altering decisions for our patients while recognizing our personal shortcomings, but we never were taught how to live with the consequences our patients must bear when we fail them.

Prayer 79 (June 6, 2020)
Jesus, Son of God and king of all, savior of my soul, I'm filled with worries about my ability to do my job, my health, my place in the world, and the safety of my loved ones.
The struggles of life sometimes seem overwhelming.
You promised to take on our burdens, Lord Jesus, and I accept.
I give myself over to you, with all my worries and anxiety.
Take them from me as you took away my sins.

Teach me to lean on you, to trust you, to know that in your ultimate victory, all my fears will prove illusory, and my pain only temporary.
Lord, do not turn your face away.
Forgive my every sin and put your mighty arms around me, for I am your child and I know you love me.

Subsequently, Javier, one of our "can-do" line-team therapists (experts at putting in difficult IV lines), started putting dialysis lines in proned patients so that we would not have to risk another death such as Lambert's. I had never heard of anyone doing something like this before. It required "Javi" to perform the procedure bent-over under the bed, doing every step of the procedure upside-down and backward. As the months went by, Javi was repeatedly called to place dialysis lines in proned patients since many of our Covid pneumonia patients eventually went into kidney failure. He never failed to get a line, and we never lost another patient supinating them to place a dialysis line.

Prayer 80 (June 7, 2020)
Sovereign Lord, bless your people, your flock.
Give your peace, mercy and love to your servants, the sheep of your fold, so that we can be united in the bond of peace and love, one body and one Spirit, in one hope of our calling, in your divine and boundless love.
Tomorrow Lord, let us be men and women and pick up our crosses, and carry them by the strength of your Holy Spirit.
[Psalm 99 abbreviated and updated]

On this day, we admitted Lin, a 92-year-old Asian man intubated in the ER due to severe Covid pneumonia. Lin was bedridden and uncommunicative due to dementia. It seemed to me that his age alone made it unlikely that he could survive. But his son pre-empted any discussion of limiting code status by going straight to our Chief Medical Officer at the time of admission and informing him that, as Lin's surrogate, he refused any discussion of DNR status. Lin would be expected to receive full life support whatever happened and without any further discussion with the doctors or nurses.

Prayer 81 (June 8, 2020)

Lord, I think you created dogs to teach us a few things.

I want to come before you with no specific requests today Lord. Just filled with joy to sit at your feet, and to gaze up at your face in rapture. No worries about the future – you got it covered.

Under your roof, I am secure; completely forgetting all my failures – they are washed away forever.

The greatest thing for me is for you to reach down and put your hand upon my head and smile at me.

I don't try to figure out why you love me, I just know you do and I accept it.

June 2020. *Jem (foreground) and Einstein (background) waiting for me to get home at dusk.*

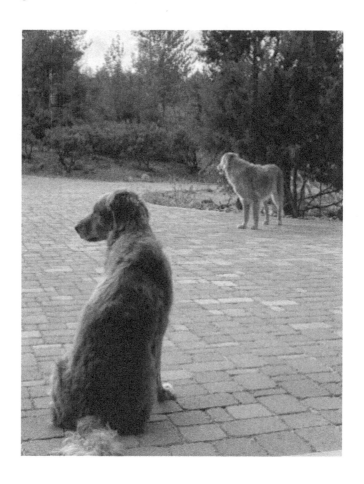

Prayer 82 (June 9, 2020)
Jesus is my shepherd – What else could I ever want?
He bestows me his peace on Earth and prepares a place for me in Heaven.
His Holy Spirit keeps me righteous.
No matter what mistakes I make, no matter what earthly catastrophe befalls, I shall not be afraid for he is by my side.
[Adaptation of Psalm 23, part 1]

A nearby hospital experienced a Covid outbreak in a *non-Covid* hospital ward for orthopedic patients. Seventeen healthcare workers were infected, including a young physician who became critically ill, requiring admission to the ICU. This confirmed something that I had been thinking about for the past few weeks. The prevalence of Covid in our state was so high now that even someone who came in with a broken toenail might well have Covid. Given our high-level vigilance inside the Covid cohort zone, the risk of catching Covid might actually be higher *outside* it! Now we couldn't let our guard down *anywhere* in the hospital.

Prayer 83 (June 10, 2020)
Father we praise you for using us to bring joy to your Son.
In the midst of all the struggles and discouragement we face, continue transforming us into servants of good courage.
Lead us by your Holy Spirit to find rest in the promises you revealed to us in your word.
Prepare us for the day when you will judge an account of all our works and offenses.
We don't deserve your grace, and we cannot begin to express our gratitude for nailing our guilt upon the cross.
We long to experience the moment when you will declare to us, "Well done good and faithful servant, enter into the joy of your master."
[Taken loosely from 2 Corinthians 5 and directly from Matthew 25:23]

Prayer 84 (June 11, 2020)
My path is clear.
He lifted me up out of the pit, healed all my shortcomings, and awarded me the highest honor, which even the angels envy – he called me his son, his brother!
Surely goodness and mercy will follow me all the days of my life and I will dwell in the house of the Lord forever!
[Adaptation of Psalm 23, part 2]

Lin, the 92-year-old man with dementia, surprised us all, improving to the point that we successfully extubated him – one of the easiest and quickest recoveries we ever saw from Covid pneumonia requiring mechanical ventilation. His benign course was at odds with data (and common sense) that showed a strong correlation between advanced age and fatal outcomes.

The same day, we received the sad news that Anderson, the stubborn 27-year-old Navajo man whom we had transferred for ECMO, had passed away despite having received the highest level of life support available. A grim reminder: statistics that apply to large populations don't always predict what will happen to an individual patient. Anderson left a wife and three children, remembered in my prayers.

Prayer 85 (June 12, 2020)
I knew yesterday that today was going to be tough.
I'm a slow learner Lord, but each day of my life that you get me through in one piece slowly gets it through my thick skull that you have my back. And that whatever materially happens, the faith you have freely given me is sufficient to get me through.
I'm so weak, I will forget this again tomorrow and you'll have to show me all over again, in your infinite patience and mercy.
I am only worthy of your loving-kindness on account of Christ's blood.
Thanks for never giving up on me Lord and please get me through the rest of this day.

On this day, 13 of 25 patients in our ICU had Covid pneumonia. We were approaching the limit of the number of patients we could safely take care of. I arrived at work at 6 am that day and left for home after 8 pm. Although Covid cases were declining in much of the United States, Arizona was in the midst of a rapid upward surge. On this single day in June, there were over 1300 patients newly hospitalized for Covid in our state. We didn't know it at the time, but that number would grow to over 3500 hospitalizations and 100 deaths *per day* within the following four weeks, making Arizona the state with the highest per-capita Covid attack rate in the U.S.

Today, I admitted Clayton, a 50-year-old man who was sick with Covid at home for 16 days, unsuccessfully treated with hydroxychloroquine, azithromycin, and penicillin (none of which have any benefit in Covid). By the time he reached our ER, his pneumonia was so severe he required immediate intubation. Clayton had no past medical history and no risk factors for severe Covid except that he was a bit overweight. But he was already in the early stages of kidney failure and would require dialysis soon after his arrival in the ICU. We started him on blood thinners to prevent blood clots in the veins of his legs and the lungs – a potentially life-threatening complication that was being reported in association with Covid pneumonia. He was enlisted in a research trial of convalescent plasma.

His wife Estelle asked if there was any way she could come see him, and I was sorry to have to tell her no. From March through September 2020, our ICU had a strict no-visitation policy. Clayton wouldn't see his wife, son, or daughter until he left the hospital, a shell of his former self, 35 days later.

Prayer 86 (June 13, 2020)

I lift up my eyes to the mountain – where does my help come from?
My help comes from the Lord, the maker of Heaven and Earth.
He will not let my foot slip. He who watches over me never sleeps.
The Lord is the shade at my right hand; the sun will not harm me by day, nor the moon by night.
The Lord will keep me from all harm – he safeguards my soul.
The Lord defends me, coming and going, both now and forevermore. [From Psalm 121]

I left home for work at 5:30 and arrived by 6 am. I had several reasons for starting the day early – it greatly reduced the chances of ever being late for the official start of my shift at

7 am, it gave me a head start on my work (which had become a practical necessity), and I occasionally got to see a spectacular sunrise. The cafeteria opened at six, and I could grab a coffee and ask Yuri to make me a breakfast sandwich before heading up to the unit.

My next stop was the ICU locker room, where I grabbed clean scrubs and put them on over my work clothes. Then I headed out to the wards to establish my computer workstation for the day. Pre-Covid, we freely shared a large number of computer workstations at every desk in the ICU. But the keyboards were now suspected as a potential source of Covid contact exposure and I had begun to choose one location to do all my charting all day, cleaning the entire workstation, keyboard and mouse with antiviral wipes and posting a dated and autographed sign indicating that I was using it, and asking others to keep off. Next, I printed my patient list and looked over as many of the morning labs and X-rays as I could before 7 am, when we did the check-in. By 7:30 or so, after we were done with that, the night shift headed home and I started seeing patients.

I put on my P100 mask, adjusting the four straps until the seal was perfect and headed to the Covid cohort zone to see patients one by one. I left my P100 on in between patients, washing my hands and changing out my gown and gloves before entering each room. The gowns we had at the time were made of shiny, blue plastic; thin-ply and easily torn, the material was cheaper than that used for garbage bags and I sweated like crazy in them. An isolation stethoscope hung inside each patient room. It was hard to hear much with those cheap devices, which seemed to be more of a prop than an actual medical instrument.

Once I had seen as many Covid patients as I could (limited by how much individual patient information I could store in my short-term memory and how long I could stand wearing my P100), I would don clean gloves, wash the outside of my P100 with an antiviral wipe while still wearing it, then take all my Covid PPE off, put a surgical mask on, and document all my findings in the EMR. Seeing Covid patients was interrupted frequently and for a number of reasons – pages, texts, consults, and acute deterioration of existing patients. Untimely interruptions, such as a pager going off while in the room of a Covid patient, required the removal of all Covid PPE. We were putting PPE on and taking it off at an incredible rate each day, drastically impacting our efficiency and rapidly filling our contamination waste bins. I don't know how the hospital kept us stocked up, but they had it down by this point.

This process was repeated until all the existing patients were seen. After a quick lunch, I started seeing the new admissions and existing patients who were deteriorating, following up on all X-rays and labs, responding to nursing concerns and calling families that requested information. Seven pm check-out came around all too soon most days. I commonly didn't get home until after 8 pm.

Prayer 87 (June 14, 2020)
I tried just quietly listening today for my prayer. I heard this thought/image:
There's war all around us.
Titanic, uncontrollable forces threaten us.
All we have to protect us is our faith and all we can do to fight back is love one another in our every day interactions.
But weak as we are individually, our actions are incredibly powerful bound together by the Holy Spirit.
We can and will win this war.
God has decreed light will conquer darkness in his holy name.
Thank you Lord for sending this encouragement.
We are stronger than the enemy wants us to believe!

Clayton's O2 sat worsened. We had to prone him and heavily sedate and paralyze him to get him in synchrony with the ventilator. His kidneys completely failed, requiring continuous dialysis. His blood glucose level consistently rose into the 300 range (100 being normal), at least partially due to dexamethasone. He had now become – *and as it turns out, would remain* – an insulin-requiring diabetic.

Prayer 88 (June 15, 2020)
Lord, thanks for getting us through this day – another opportunity to bring your kingdom a little bit closer to Earth.
I hope I don't regret asking Lord, but use me tomorrow.
Give me a job to do and give me the strength to do it, whatever it is.
Our purpose on Earth is to learn to do your will.
Let us find peace and happiness in that, whatever our material circumstances.
The best thing in life is knowing we are your sons and daughters –
we have a purpose and an all-powerful Father who loves us.

Prayer 89 (June 16, 2020)
Let the words of my mouth and the meditations of my heart be acceptable in your sight, O Lord.
Help me tune out worldly influences which would lead me to waste my life.
Let your Holy Spirit guide me in thought and action.
Grant me the grace to hear your word.
Soften my heart so that I can be directed only by your truth.
I ask this in the holy name of your son, my savior Jesus Christ

Preliminary results of the RECOVERY trial were released on June 16. This study enrolled over 6000 patients in the strongest experiment design: the randomized controlled trial. RECOVERY showed that dexamethasone, a widely available and relatively inexpensive steroid drug, reduced death by one-fifth in Covid patients requiring oxygen, and by one-third in those requiring mechanical ventilation. This translates to one life saved for every eight intubated patients, the most effective treatment for severe Covid pneumonia even to this day. We learned about these preliminary results via social media in the morning and by lunchtime, all our ICU Covid pneumonia patients, including Clayton, were receiving dexamethasone.

Later that same day, we admitted Vincenzo, a 63-year-old man who presented with fever, diarrhea and cough. Vincenzo had been unsuccessfully treated with atovaquone, an antifungal agent used for AIDS-related pneumonia, being given for Covid despite the lack of any convincing data it worked. Per our normal practice on admission, we asked Vincenzo what he would want us to do if he were to worsen to the point of requiring life support. Vincenzo said he would not want life support even if it meant he would die without it. "I would rather die" were his final (and hopefully non-prophetic) words.

Prayer 90 (June 17, 2020)
Lord, we can feel the promise of the Holy Spirit in our souls.
But we groan inwardly with impatience as we eagerly wait to be delivered, for our bodies to be renewed, and to join Jesus under your roof in Heaven. For in this hope we were saved.
It's hard to imagine this bright future from where we now stand, but you gave us the great gift of faith so that we can patiently hope for that which we cannot see.
And you also gave us your Holy Spirit to help us in our weakness. For we do not even know how to pray, but your Holy Spirit himself prays for us with emotions too deep for human words. And the one who searches our hearts knows the mind of the Spirit, interceding for us according to the will of God.
And you also gave us the assurance that, for those who love God, all things work together for good, for we are called according to your good purpose.
[Interpretation of Romans 8:22-30]

In Arizona, we experience a prominent annual variation in the patient census (the number of patients currently under our care in the ICU). Winter was busier due to "snowbirds" who travel to Arizona to escape the cold weather back east. So although our average ICU census was 16 patients, there were typically far fewer in the summer.

This summer was a major exception. We were admitting new Covid patients every day now, and most were "rocks" (patients that require a long ICU stay, whether they recover or die). Our census relentlessly rose into the mid-twenties – the maximum number we previously believed to be safe. An escalation from 16 to 24 patients represents a 50% increase over our average workload. On top of sheer numbers, Covid patients were significantly sicker than our usual patients. There was no reserve ICU physician staff to call in; we just each had to individually pick up our pace.

Our group met via Zoom to discuss our maximal capacity in relation to the hospital's "surge plan" – a policy to deal with the possibility that Covid patients would eventually overwhelm our capacity. I noticed something funny during the meeting. *Am I really seeing what I think I'm seeing?* Mayfield was on-video with a glass of red wine in his hand (he was off-duty) and he took a sip every single time anyone uttered the words "surge plan." At this rate, he would be happily bombed by the end of the meeting!

After thoughtful debate, Mayfield's wine consumption notwithstanding, our group decided we could safely see no more than 26 patients per day. To put this number in perspective, we had only reached a census as high as 26 *once* in all of 2019. Subsequently, as part of the surge plan, various groups of physicians volunteered to help out if our census exceeded 26, including the trauma/ICU surgeons (our closest colleagues), ER physicians and anesthesiologists. As the weeks passed, we found that we could stretch far beyond the limits of our ability as we perceived it back in June 2020. But for the purposes of tracking how busy we were soon to get, I henceforth counted 26 ICU patients as 100% "maximum safe census" as a metric of how busy our service later became.

Prayer 91 (June 18, 2020)
Preserve me, O Lord, for in you I take refuge.
You are my Lord – I have no good apart from you.
I bless the Lord, who gives me counsel.
I have set the Lord always before me.

Because he is by my side, I shall not be shaken.
You have made known to me the path of life.
I find everlasting happiness and peace in your presence.
Keep me by your side. [From Psalm 16]

The state health department had taken command of Covid patient triage from outlying hospitals to coordinate the utilization of healthcare resources during the surge. Although it was clear from our standpoint that "capacity" should be defined by the number of available nurses and doctors, the state defined it based on the number of licensed ICU rooms in the hospital building. Through an unfortunate historical quirk, our hospital had an exceptionally large number of unused rooms licensed as ICU rooms, although we had no extra doctors or nurses to staff them. The state health department considered that *our* problem. Therefore, we were each expected to stretch our personal capacity to twice, even three times, normal levels to keep up with transfers. We griped a little bit about being called to "give 110%", but there was never any question that we would take care of whatever patients came our way to the best of our ability.

Prayer 92 (June 19, 2020)
Dear Lord I pray for America.
Give our leaders wisdom and integrity to lead us in the right direction, so that their decisions will be based on loving and serving each other, as the Father commanded.
As troubles mount, I pray the light of your love will shine on our land and peace reign in our nation.
Protect us from those who seek our downfall.
I thank you that I was born in America and I'm grateful to be a citizen of this great nation.
But Lord, help us to be better – to be everything that you would have us be, to love each other as a nation that embraces your Holy Spirit and acknowledges you as Lord!

Prayer 93 (June 20, 2020)

In the olden days Lord, you would sometimes command your people Israel to war, and when they obeyed, their enemies were destroyed, no matter the odds. Complete victory always followed obedience.
Now, we are your adopted sons and daughters, warriors at your command. I sometimes worry that we are weak warriors Lord – not as strong as our moms and dads were – but then I remember that doesn't matter to you.
We don't have to be strong, we just have to obey.
Lord open our ears and soften our hearts to your commands so that we can act on Earth in your name and never know defeat.

Our ICU census was now 23, 16 with Covid pneumonia. Clayton was making no progress despite dexamethasone, mechanical ventilation, dialysis and an insulin infusion. His glucose levels remained at levels only seen in severe insulin-dependent diabetes.

Vincenzo had also badly deteriorated and was no longer able to communicate. His wife and daughter now became his surrogate legal decision-makers. Although they knew that he didn't want life support, they reversed his DNR and asked us to do everything possible to save him. It was with some moral distress that we intubated Vincenzo. Within the next 24 hours, he was on 100% oxygen, in a proning bed, on pressors (life support drugs that maintain adequate blood pressure) and going into renal failure. It looked like we had made a grave ethical mistake together.

Prayer 94 (June 21, 2020, Father's Day)
"I am the bread of life; whoever comes to me shall not hunger, and whoever believes in me shall never thirst."

Dear heavenly father, just when I come to the point of doubt, exhaustion and fearfulness, you lift me up.
You bring me out of the depths and draw me close to your heart.
You have renewed my strength like an eagle's wings today, Lord.
Our faith is being built on all that you have provided for us in

Christ. Help us to carry forward with that today.

Thank you for being our father and helping us to remember what a father should be.

Thank you for my band of brothers; many of us are fathers trying to emulate you. Please bless them.

[Happy Fathers Day, inspired by John 6:35]

Prayer 95 (June 22, 2020)

Lord, I'm always worried about tomorrow. But you told us not to worry, just ask the Father for any good thing in your name and he will give it.

We cry out to you regarding all who are now sick and we trust that you hear us and will answer our prayers according to your will. We're not going to stop!

Praise your holy name Lord, your loving-kindness, and your great mercy.

You are the "Model Dad" that we strive to imitate in our small way, through the power of your Holy Spirit.

We thank you for our families Lord, please keep blessing and protecting them.

It was recognized that Covid caused a derangement in blood coagulation that increased the risk of blood clots by about 5-10 times. So our Covid patients routinely received precautionary low-dose blood thinners to prevent blood clots in their legs, which could dislodge and dangerously impact their lungs (a life-threatening event called pulmonary embolism). But Clayton developed a blood clot in his legs *despite this precaution,* and we had to ramp him up to full-dose blood thinners.

Prayer 96 (June 23, 2020)

Jesus – our creator and savior.

Our shepherd, our healer, our friend and brother, who commands the Heavens and this little dust-speck we live on.

Master of past, present and future – bless the brief moment your children call "tomorrow."

We will need you to bless our bodies with health.
We will need you to provide air for us to breathe, water to drink and food.
We will need you to restrain Satan from destroying us as he ravenously desires.
We will need your Holy Spirit to guide our hearts and our minds in all the challenges we will face.
We will need your strength to resist temptation.
We will need wisdom and courage that comes from your gift of faith.
Let us bring glory to you by loving our brothers and sisters, today and tomorrow in your holy name.

For the past week, the "Bush Fire" had been burning northeast of Phoenix in the Tonto National Forest. Started by a car that caught fire and pulled off the road over some dry grass, the wildfire thrived in triple-digit Arizona heat, burning over 300 square miles of chaparral and desert. Smoke from the fire was visible from the porch of our home in Phoenix. On our trips up to Payson, we drove past thousands of charred ocotillos, palo verdes and saguaro cacti – some of the later were centuries old, now burned to cinders. It crossed my mind that we wouldn't live long enough to see the regrowth of this habitat. On this day, our brave firefighters had finally gotten the fire under control. By God's grace, they all returned home safe to their families.

Prayer 97 (June 24, 2020)
My wife and I are up in Payson and the air is clear of smoke.
Lord you restore all things according to your ways.
Thank you for always being there to clean up our messes.
God, incline your ear to us; hear our prayers.
Show your steadfast love, O Savior of those who seek refuge.
Hide us in the shadow of your wings tonight while we sleep, and awaken us tomorrow morning full of your Holy Spirit.
[Adaptation of Psalm 17]

Our ICU census was 28 today, 21 with Covid pneumonia. One of the busiest days so far in the history of our group.

Prayer 98 (June 25, 2020)
Lord, we thank you and we praise you.
It's hard for me to keep in mind, but so comforting to know that you love our children far more than we ever can, and that any good thing that we ask for them, in your name, will be given.
Your will defines goodness.
Lord, just say the word and your word will take form.
Bless the doctors and nurses so that they can be part of your miraculous healing.
Bless our patients and their families – please give them some rest and peace knowing that your mighty and loving arms have each of them covered.

Vincenzo was not responding to treatment. Our palliative care team met with his wife and daughters to discuss withdrawing life support and focusing on comfort care. Vincenzo's family wanted to continue aggressive care but agreed that we should not escalate to CPR if Vincenzo coded. If that happened, we would finally honor Vincenzo's expressed wishes and let him go.

Prayer 99 (June 26, 2020)
I asked the Lord how to pray today and I heard, "Pray for our young adult children."
Lord, everything that our kids need the most right now – courage, steadfastness, perseverance, and hope – can only be theirs through faith in you.
I haven't been the best spiritual father to my kids, but you never needed me to perform well to claim my kids as your own.
Take our children under your wing.
Say the word and count them among your flock.
Then every measure of blessing will be theirs through your grace.
And help us, flawed earthly moms and dads, play some part in

your good plan for them. Thank you Father for hearing our prayer.

Clayton began vomiting-up blood. This was at least partially due to the high-dose blood thinners he was receiving for the blood clot in his leg. We couldn't win no matter which way we turned, but it's usually best to comply with the old saying: *first, do no harm*. We discontinued blood thinners and supined Clayton long enough for a gastrointestinal specialist to cauterize the ulcer in his stomach through an endoscope passed down his throat.

Prayer 100 (June 27, 2020)
Lord, a hundred days ago, my brothers and I promised to share a hundred daily prayers to get us through the end of the Covid pandemic. You must have smiled at my foolishness.
Here we are in Arizona a hundred days later, and we are on the upslope of the worst Covid surge in the world.
Guess we aren't done praying yet.
I can't believe what you carried us through already Lord.
All praise and thanks to you!
You've taught us so much while protecting us from disaster.
You poured down your grace in the form of faith upon us all.
I'm looking around this ICU full to the rafters, with total confidence in you and no worry anymore.
My God is an awesome God! He is alive.
He is carrying me through life, and nothing can stop him!

My bible study brothers and I talked it over and decided it didn't make any sense to stop at 100 prayers while we were still in the midst of catastrophe. [*From this point forward, I eased up on the self-imposed requirement to share a prayer every single day, so readers will notice the prayers are more spaced out in time from here on out.*]

Prayer 101 (June 28, 2020)
How abundant is your goodness, which you have worked for those

who take refuge in you. (Psalm 31:19)

Dear Lord, thank you for being with us.
We know you are faithful.
You never lead us into a place where you will not also lead us out.
Help us to know that on the other side of the desert is the promised
land. We praise you for your radiant glory that is revealed through
your son Jesus.
We believe, Lord, help us in our unbelief! (Mark 9:24)
[Offered by Mike U.]

Ten of our Covid pneumonia patients were now in proning beds. I could see such patients for days on end without ever speaking to them, without even *seeing them*; as they became dehumanized inside the mechanism of the proning bed. The practical work of the day could be completed by merely focusing on their vitals, laboratory values, chest X-ray, and a set of ventilator settings to be adjusted.

One day I caught myself collecting data for my notes in the room of a proned patient, and I realized I didn't know their name. Like all proned patients, he, *she? – the patient's gender was in no way apparent* – was under heavy sedation, unable to communicate, even by nodding their head or raising an eyebrow. I went to the head of the bed, bent-over almost double at the waist to see under the proning bed. I noticed a partially dried pool of nasal secretions had leaked out onto the floor. I looked back up at the patient's inverted face, grossly swollen and distorted by the prolonged effects of gravity, and I wasn't sure I would be able to recognize them, even if I knew who they were. I straightened up; no other part of their body was visible without partially dissembling the bed. I didn't have time for that. I snaked my gloved fingers between two of the thick foam pads until I touched a part of the patient's back somewhere, just to have made physical contact with them somewhere.

Prayer 102 (June 29, 2020)

The Lord is my rock, my fortress and my deliverer, in whom I take refuge.
I call upon the Lord who is worthy to be praised, and I am saved from all adversity.
The torrents of death encompassed me, the cords of hell entangled me!
In my distress I called upon my God; I cried for help.
And from his temple he heard my voice; my cry reached his ears.
Then the Earth reeled and the foundations of the mountains trembled. The Lord also thundered in the Heavens, and the Most High uttered his voice.
He sent from on high. He took me.
He drew me out of deep waters and brought me into a broad place.
He rescued me because he delighted in me.
[Adaptation of Psalm 18]

On this day, we took care of 34 patients (140% of our previous maximum safe census), 31 of whom were on life support due to Covid pneumonia.

It was so busy now that something had to give. My daily patient care routine, developed over 34 years of practice, had become irrelevant, and in any case, could no longer be maintained. Part of that routine was listening to the patient's heart and lungs each day. We did this in the Covid cohort unit, which was now overflowing to fill the majority of our ICU beds, using disposable "isolation stethoscopes" to prevent spreading Covid room-to-room with our personal stethoscopes. However, it was hard to hear much of anything with isolation stethoscopes, little better than the ones a kid might play doctor with. I had been cleaning the earpieces of the isolation stethoscopes with alcohol before each use but couldn't wait to let them dry before sticking them in my ears. Now, the repeated exposure to alcohol had damaged my left eardrum and it painfully popped every time I swallowed. I finally decided to stop examining Covid pneumonia patients with the isolation stethoscopes altogether, concentrating instead on visual and tactile examination. It seemed like professional sacrilege to me, but I had to be realistic.

Prayer 103 (June 30, 2020)
I wonder how tomorrow might be different than any other day.
Will I just get through the day, reacting to whatever worldly events occur, or will I exercise my faith and change the course of events according to God's will?
Lord, don't let me stagnate. Let me grow in faith.
Let my prayers lead me closer to you.
Reveal your deep wisdom to me when I read your book.
Reveal to me the job you have for me in relation to each person I meet.
Make me a clean vessel for your Holy Spirit.
Make tomorrow meaningful in your holy name.

We were able to take Clayton out of the proning bed. Having been face-down for more than two weeks, gravity had grossly distorted his facial features. His entire head was swollen, and he had black pressure sores on his cheeks and chin and under his nose, where the endotracheal tube had been pressing. We tried to reduce his sedation so that he could start the process of breathing on his own again, but he became severely agitated. He developed violent shaking chills (that often presage blood stream infections) followed by a 103-degree fever spike. I re-sedated him, cultured his blood and respiratory secretions and started antibiotics. Respiratory cultures later grew a bacteria called Stenotrophomonas, in this case likely representing secondary bacterial pneumonia.

[It is difficult to definitively diagnose secondary bacterial pneumonia in patients who already have Covid pneumonia since they have overlapping clinical and radiographic findings. Once a patient is intubated, it's just a matter of 4-5 days before their respiratory secretions become overgrown with bacteria, which treat the ETT like a condominium. Its often impossible to know for sure whether these bacteria are merely colonizing the ETT or taking

advantage of exhausted host defenses to invade the lungs. We took our best-educated guess – if the patient suddenly deteriorated as Clayton did, and we found a new bacteria in their sputum, we treated it as secondary bacterial pneumonia.]

Prayer 104 (July 1, 2020)
Lord, we are increasingly bombarded by harmful voices – politicians, news media, Twitter, Facebook, etc. – threatening to drown out your gentle wisdom and turn our hearts cold and fearful.
Lord, help me ignore them.
But let me hear, and let my mind dwell on, whatever is true, whatever is noble, right, pure, lovely, whatever is admirable, excellent or praiseworthy.
Lord, fill my mind with your Good News!
And may your peace, which surpasses all understanding, guard our hearts and minds. [Derived from Philippians 4:6-9]

I saw 20 patients, 17 with Covid, over the course of the day – the most I had ever seen in a 12-hour shift. If you do the math, it allows just over a half hour per patient, inclusive of all bedside care, data assimilation, charting, order writing, family communication, "putting out fires" (taking care of myriad changes in patients clinical condition) and interruptions for admissions, codes and procedures. This demanded unrelenting work-pace and efficiency such as never before required of us over sustained periods of time. This was a short-lived record, repeatedly broken in the coming months.

Prayer 105 (July 2, 2020)
Lord, I know someday, when we are with you in Heaven, our life on Earth may not seem so great.
But right now, today, I love the life you made for me; the blessings you have showered on me: my health, my loving and beautiful and faithful wife, my wonderfully talented and challenging children, my brothers in Christ, my friends, the great people I work with, the roof over my head, the wondrous and beautiful world you

made for us, the growth-provoking challenges that come our way each day, our loyal and goofy dogs, the great book I'm reading, the patches of saguaros that survived the Arizona wildfire.
It's all down to you, my Lord.
Thank you so much for life. The chance to be blessed by you.
And to be able to be dumb and make mistakes, even purposely doing bad things at times, yet having been gifted with faith, by which we are made righteous through your Son's holy blood, we are promised eternity in paradise with you.
How could I not be happy?
How you must love us to invent such a lopsided deal in our favor!
Thank you, my Lord and my Savior!

My partner Mayfield was seeing Mario, a 42-year-old man with Covid pneumonia who required semi-emergent intubation. As Mayfield got the intubation equipment and sedation medications together, I noticed nurse Samantha in the room, bent over by the head of the bed, shouting at Mario to be heard through her P100 and over the hiss of his BiPAP mask. She then held a cellphone up to his face briefly, and I saw Mario looking into it and shouting, although I couldn't make him out. Then Mayfield entered the room, sedated and intubated Mario.

Later, I learned that Sam and the other nurses had been assisting many of the Covid patients to record video messages for their families before intubation, cognizant that some would never get to see their loved ones again and these might well be the last words their families would ever hear from them.

A few days later, I walked by Mario's room and noticed a new Covid patient in the bed. Mario was gone – *deceased* – his bed having been immediately taken by another. His cellphone and final video message would be returned to his family, along with whatever other personal belongings he might have brought to the hospital.

Prayer 106 (July 3, 2020)

O God, from my youth you have taught me, and I proclaim your wonderous deeds.
Even to old age and gray hairs, God, do not forsake me until I proclaim your might to another generation – your power to all those to come.
Your righteousness, God reaches to the high Heavens.
You have done great things God. Who is like you?
You've seen me through many troubles and calamities and will revive me again even from the depths of the Earth.
My lips will shout for joy when I sing my praises to you!
[From Psalm 71]

Prayer 107 (July 5, 2020)
Lord Jesus Christ, the Son of God, have mercy on me, a sinner.
At the name of Jesus, let every knee bend, in Heaven, on Earth, and beneath the Earth, and let every tongue confess that Jesus is Lord, to the glory of God the Father.
["The Jesus Prayer," Luke 18:13 and Philippians 2:9-11]

This was a very bad day for Vincenzo. The cuff that seals the endotracheal tube in Vincenzo's throat ruptured, causing catastrophic loss of the pressure inflating his lungs. While Joyce was performing an ETT exchange, his right lung ruptured and collapsed. He was "no code" but never technically lost his pulse, so Joyce fought aggressively to keep him alive, starting pressors and performing emergency bedside chest tube surgery to get his lung re-inflated. He just barely survived this double attempt on his life and seemed to be at the absolute end of his rope. His body had wasted away despite tube feedings, apparently unable to utilize the nutrition he was receiving. The metabolic demands of his fight to stay alive were burning through his last reserves. His blood pressure was barely compatible with life despite multiple pressors, and he was comatose on sedatives and narcotics required to keep him from fighting the vent. This couldn't possibly go on much longer.

Prayer 108 (July 6, 2020)

Lord, it was 1982 when I said one of the most important prayers of my life: sitting on the grass outside Apache dorm at the University of Arizona, thinking I would never meet the right girl, I asked you to send me the partner I was supposed to spend the rest of my life with. And shortly thereafter, I met Jean.

We are celebrating our 36th anniversary today, and through many ups and downs (mostly ups) I have never doubted she was your answer to my prayer.
You know what an angel your daughter Jean is.
I can't believe you entrusted her to me.
Today, we invited the kids over for our anniversary and our whole family is in the kitchen, cooking and joking around together.
Thank you Lord Jesus for answering my prayer in this way.
Please look into my heart Lord to feel the extent of my gratitude, which these clumsy words can barely express.
My Lord – the hearer of my prayers! All praise and thanks to you!

It seems an abrupt digression to leave Vincenzo hanging and talk about my home life, but the two were intricately connected. I don't think I could do my job if it wasn't for the support I receive from my wife.

Jean is the most selfless person I know, always putting others before herself. Smarter than me – *though somehow I ended up the doctor of the family.* It had taken me most of 36 years to start taking her sparingly-given advice, which almost always turns out to be right. Jean has an honest and easy laugh – important to a guy with a corny sense of humor like me. She is faithful. I have always trusted her implicitly and she has never once let me down in regard to any important matter.

And here's something I think about Jean some mornings as I leave for work and kiss her goodbye, saying, "Love you, sweety – see you tonight." *I think she is Jesus' most beloved daughter, yet the Most Intimidating Father in the universe gave me his permission to marry her! He entrusted the one he loves to my care!* That is a responsibility I'm unlikely to mess up.

Prayer 109 (July 7, 2020)
Jesus, through your sacrifice, we obtained access by faith into God's grace, in which we stand.
We rejoice in hope of the glory of God, and with your Holy Spirit, we can even rejoice in our suffering, knowing that suffering produces endurance, endurance produces character, and character produces hope.
And hope does not put us to shame because God's love has been poured into our hearts through the Holy Spirit who has been given to us!
For this light momentary affliction is preparing for us an eternal weight of glory beyond all comparison, as we look not to the things that are seen but to the things that are unseen.
All glory to you, in Heaven and on Earth, forever.
[From Romans 5 and 2 Corinthians 4]

On July 8, 2020, as Vincenzo and twenty other Covid pneumonia patients were fighting for their lives in our ICU, the New York Times reported that Arizona had the highest per capita Covid attack rate of any state or country in the world. However, outside the hospital, I commonly encountered people deriding the "scam-demic" – vocally expressing their unwillingness to wear a mask in public. As I walked down the bustling hallway of our ICU, passing room after room of Covid patients on ventilators struggling to barely survive, I wished I could take these Covid-deniers on a quick tour.

Prayer 110 (July 10, 2020)
God, if you are for us, who can be against us?
You gave your only Son for our salvation!
How can you not also graciously give us all things?

Who shall bring any charge against those you chose?
You are the one who justifies.
No one can condemn us when Jesus Christ died and was raised on our behalf and is at your right hand interceding for us.

Who shall separate us from the love of Christ?
Shall tribulation, distress, persecution or adversity? No!

In all these things, you have made us conquerors Jesus, through
your love, and now we are certain that neither death nor life, nor
angels nor rulers, nor things present or yet to come, nor height nor
depth nor anything else in all creation can separate us from your
love – Christ Jesus our Lord!
[From Romans 8:31-39]

On this date, three years ago, Dr. Dominick Novak, my mentor and the closest thing I had to a big brother, passed away. I took a moment this morning to remember Dom. I sure could use some inspiration from him about now.

I met Dom when I was a fourth-year medical student in 1985. He was the best doctor I had ever met at that early point of my career, and my high opinion of him stood-up over the 30 years our practices overlapped. He had a rare combination of intelligence, decisiveness (a touch of cockiness at times), blunt honesty, deep compassion for the suffering of others, commitment to his profession, and wicked good humor. Thinking about Dom reminded me of the story of one of our greatest shared experiences: Inez's story.

Inez was a 34-year-old firefighter who presented to our ICU in 2004. She experienced an unrecognized bowel perforation as a complication of an appendectomy surgery. Sent home after surgery, she was so tough that she initially thought the extreme abdominal pain she was experiencing was "normal" after surgery. But the breach of containment of bacteria residing in her bowels soon sent Inez into septic shock – a state in which the infection overwhelmed her immune system and caused her organs to shut down. She required emergency surgery to repair her bowel, and post-op, four pressor infusions were barely holding her blood pressure compatible with life. She was on the highest levels of ventilator support available, in a coma and in kidney failure. On her fourth ICU day, her surgical wound dehisced (opened back up) and stool issued forth from the contaminated wound. The internal surgical bowel anastomosis had disintegrated.

Dom and I met with Inez's husband, Nathaniel, also a firefighter, to give him that horrible news. Nate was 6'6" and 280 pounds of rock-solid intimidating muscle – *you could easily imagine him carrying an unconscious victim out of a burning building slung over his huge shoulder like a rag doll.* A doctor's mistake had put his wife's life in extreme jeopardy, and he wasn't in any mood to trust or bandy words with any other doctor. He told us, somewhat menacingly, to give it to him straight.

Dom did all the talking. In a nutshell, he *guaranteed* Nate that Inez was going to make it.

I was flabbergasted, although I tried not to let it show. Dom *knew* that Inez's objective chances of survival were close to zero. But he wasn't being stupid or cocky – he was making a commitment to Inez and Nate, and to himself and *I guess to me too*, that we were going to move Heaven and Earth to get Inez through. And over the next three months, that's what we did. We made it personal. Dom and I provided Inez with the best possible round-the-clock care that we could. Even after Inez left the ICU for a rehab center across the street, we frequently visited her, several times readmitting her to the hospital for a long list of complications that seemed like they would never end. But the complications *did* end, and eventually Inez made a complete recovery. That blind-faith commitment to her care paid off.

One memorable spiritual event happened in the first week of Inez's illness that changed the course of my career. Inez's mom Marta was holding vigil at her bedside daily, praying the Rosary and begging Jesus to heal her daughter. One day as she prayed, I walked into the room. I didn't know it at the time, but Inez later told me, somewhat to my embarrassment, that with my long hair and beard and backlit by the sun shining through the window behind me, Marta at first thought I was a visitation of Jesus himself in answer to her prayer!

She was no-doubt disappointed to meet the real me. But after Inez told me the story, I felt like I had something to live-up-to. I couldn't *completely* disappoint that faithful woman. *Who knows, maybe Jesus set me up.* I began praying each day with Inez, Marta and Nate; and kept it up to some extent even after they left the hospital. I prayed with them over the phone that Christmas from Chicago, where I was spending time with my family. In all the years since we took care of Inez, I never lost touch with her and Nate and we still text prayer requests back and forth to each other from time to time.

Inez comes back into this story in the coming months. And Dom returns in my memories to help me though several difficult junctures ahead, as he did on this day.

Prayer 111 (July 12, 2020, for the families of Covid patients)
Lord Jesus – families are losing loved ones without being at their bedside, without being able to hold their hand, or pray with them at the end – without being able even to have a proper funeral.
But those of us you chose to be your sons and daughters still have the ultimate consolation, knowing that you are in charge in Heaven and on Earth and nothing happens to your children aside from your plan.
Where earthly social customs are failing Lord, let your mercy and grace abound and unburden the hearts of these families.
Grant them the faith to believe: you are with them now and forever if they will only believe!

On July 13, 2020, Covid peaked in Arizona. Three thousand five hundred and seventeen patients were currently hospitalized with Covid pneumonia; 970 were in ICUs and 674 were on ventilators. Covid typically took about a month to kill, so the peak in newly reported cases in mid-July was a dire warning: things in the ICU would get worse before they got better.

I didn't know if I could take it much longer. Every patient I saw that morning had Covid pneumonia. We organized our census so that all our assigned patients were geographically grouped together for better efficiency. I went from room to room to room, seeing my patients all in a row like an assembly line. In between each, I stripped my gloves and gown, washed my hands, *decided against breaking my P100 seal to scratch my nose*, donned a new gown and gloves and entered the next room.

The patient in the next room was in a proning bed. The general purpose of entering a patient's ICU room was to talk to them if possible, examine them and check the IV infusion pumps and ventilator control panel. But this patient was deeply unconscious, invisible inside the proning bed – examining them was a physical impossibility. It would take a coordinated effort of a team of nurses a half hour to supine the patient and remove the thick blocks of padding to expose the patient to examination. This was done once a day, spaced out around the clock since the nurses were so overstretched, and never coincided with my arrival at the bedside. Even if it had, proned patients were deeply sedated, severely limiting the neurologic and other essential parts of the exam. The IV infusion pumps and ventilator control panel were *outside* the room. So there really was nothing I could do in the room. I felt like kind of an idiot standing there. I just looked around a little, then duffed my gown and gloves and moved on.

Later down the line, I saw Vincenzo. He had stabilized somewhat as we continued to ignore his request not to undergo life support. He was off pressors now, and his oxygen requirements had fallen to 60%. If he kept this up, he might be a candidate for tracheostomy soon.

Two beds down, Clayton is also now experiencing begrudgingly improving oxygenation. He had been essentially comatose due to medications. We began to reduce the cocktail of narcotics, anxiolytics and sedation drugs previously required for him to tolerate mechanical ventilation, but he was not waking up as quickly as expected.

Prayer 112 (July 13, 2020)

Heavenly Lord, you have brought me to the beginning of a new day.
As the world is renewed with the dawn, renew my heart with your
strength and purpose.
Forgive my sins of yesterday and put my feet back on your path.
This day I begin my life anew.
Shine through me so that each person I meet can feel your Holy
Spirit in my soul.
Take my hand on this journey Lord, because I can't make it on my
own. Through Christ I pray and live.

Prayer 113 (July 17, 2020)
Listen to my prayer, O Father; hear my cry!
Evening, morning and noon, I cry out in distress.
My heart is in anguish within me.
I'm shaking in fear and horror has overwhelmed me.
Oh, that I had the wings of a dove! I would fly far away; I would
hurry to my place of shelter, far from adversity.
Have mercy on me, my God, for in you I take refuge.
I take refuge in the shadow of your wings until disaster has passed.
When I am afraid, I put my trust in you.
[Adaptation of Psalm 55]

There were plans to perform a tracheostomy on Vincenzo. This was typically accomplished after about two weeks of mechanical ventilation but had gotten pushed back because we were stretched too thin to keep up with demand. "Traching" Vincenzo meant he was getting better, but it also meant surrendering the effort to get him off the ventilator any time in the near future. It had been shown that more than 90% of patients who underwent tracheostomy either passed away or remained residents of nursing homes at one-year follow-up (*not because of the tracheostomy, but because the patient was so sick that they needed one*). I wasn't a big fan of either outcome for Vincenzo.

Objective measurements of lung function showed that Vincenzo's lungs *had* slowly improved over the past ten days, but he looked like an emaciated survivor of a concentration camp. I could almost completely encircle his upper arm with a single-handed grip. His head was misshapen by the atrophy of muscles in his temples and jaws. The huge doses of narcotics and sedation drugs he had received were slowly clearing out of his system but his movements were still sluggish. I held out the middle three fingers of each of my hands in front of him. "Vincenzo – grab my fingers and give me a hard squeeze – a real bone-crusher!" He looked at his hands, my hands, furrowed his brow with concentration, grabbed my fingers and gave them a decent squeeze. I smiled at his attitude. I felt strongly motivated to spare Vincenzo the tracheostomy – a procedure he explicitly instructed us NOT to perform when he requested DNR status – and his finger-squeezing effort was enough to convince me to attempt extubation instead.

A decade-old memory came back to me, as it often did before any extubation. Dom Novak once extubated a 31-year-old man recovering from pancreatitis. When he pulled the tube, the patient immediately developed stridor – a harsh honking sound with every inhalation indicating airway obstruction. The patient's O2 sat plummeted. Dom tried to reintubate, but although he was superbly gifted at that procedure, the unexpected airway swelling was too great and the anatomy too distorted. The patient turned purple as Dom, a trauma anesthesiologist and a trauma surgeon tried unsuccessfully to re-establish the airway. This catastrophe was one of the terminal events that culminated in Dom's burnout, which I will tell you more about later.

Extubation is technically simple in most cases but has one of the highest risks of fatal complications of any procedure we perform. Almost everyone who has practiced critical care medicine for any period of time has a similar nightmare memory lurking in the back of their mind. But I stuck with my decision, either through confidence in my professional experience or stubborn stupidity; time would tell.

"Pulling the tube" always took a lot longer than expected, and the process must seem interminable to an alert patient gagging on an ETT. June, the RT, set up suctioning equipment, oxygen delivery nasal prongs and an Ambu bag (in case things went south). The tape anchoring the ETT to Vincenzo's face was gently pulled free using alcohol wipes to loosen the adhesive without tearing Vincenzo's fragile skin. June assiduously suctioned Vincenzo's mouth and lower airway. A towel was placed on Vincenzo's chest to receive the ETT. She warned him that she was going to make him cough as she deflated the ETT cuff and whatever secretions had pooled above it spilled into his airway. Then she smoothly pulled the 30 cm long ETT and 100 cm nasogastric tube out and dropped them on the towel, which was then swaddled up and set aside, almost like delivering a baby. Vincenzo looked very uncomfortable for a moment – then in great relief. His eyes were watering; he was trying to cough and spit as June commanded him to open his mouth so she could suction him again. Then she put oxygen prongs in his nose. We sat him up straighter in bed, stood back and took a look at him. He looked OK.

June: "Tell us your name!"

"Cenzo," he croaked – *he wouldn't have been able to speak if his vocal cords were obstructed.* No stridor. Vincenzo had a wet cough and June was weirdly insistent that he not swallow the secretions he brought up into his mouth, but Vincenzo stubbornly refused to open his mouth for her to suction again. He pouted like a disobedient child. I smiled – I didn't blame him; I wouldn't want that foot-long plastic suction wand jammed down my throat again, either.

Vincenzo initially seemed like he might hold his own. He was breathing at a rate of 20 breaths per minute – just a tad fast. He looked comfortable, had cleared his windpipe and his O2 sats hovered in the low 90s. But more time was needed to see if he would last. A lot of things could still go wrong. I went home that night with considerable anxiety, praying I wouldn't return in the morning again to another disaster. I didn't get much sleep that night worrying about Vincenzo.

Prayer 114 (July 18, 2020)
Oh come, let us sing to the Lord; let us make a joyful noise to the rock of our salvation!
Let us come into his presence with thanksgiving; let us make a joyful noise to him with songs of praise!
For the Lord is a great god, and a great king above all gods.
In his hand are the depths of the Earth; the heights of the mountains are his also.
The sea is his, for he made it, and his hands formed the dry land.
Oh come, let us worship and bow down; let us kneel before the Lord, Our Maker!
For he is our God, and we are the people of his hand, and the sheep of his pasture. [Psalm 95, offered by Dave T.]

I started my day at the cafeteria at 6 am. Minor disaster: the Phoenix PD beat me to the grill! There were seven uniformed officers ahead of me in line, our hospital cafeteria being one of their favorite breakfast spots. They all knew Yuri personally and were joking around with him. This was definitely going to delay the start of my workday. These hardworking women and men needed some serious calories to fuel their workday, and they didn't mess around. The officer in front of the line ordered three eggs, four pieces of bacon, two sausages, a biscuit and hash browns. Yuri gave him about eight pieces of bacon.

I remembered something I had read about the NYPD during the initial Covid surge in New York City. The police union filed a complaint because front-line police officers were not being provided masks. A spokesperson for the city called the complaint "empty rhetoric," but by the end of March, 5,600 police officers had contracted Covid – 15% of the NYPD workforce. Over the course of 2020, 221 "line-of-duty deaths" due to Covid were reported among police officers across the country.

My brief reverie broke and I decided to duck out of line, grabbing some Cheerios, a banana and coffee instead. I was anxious to check on Vincenzo, and getting up there even five minutes earlier might make a difference in how my workday went.

I popped my head into his room – Vincenzo was still holding his own! – maybe even looking a little better. At 10 am, when we were back, rounding outside Vincenzo's room with the entire ICU team, I looked in at him from the hallway outside his door and waved to him. He cracked a crooked smile and weakly waved back at me – the first discernable positive emotion he had expressed since his ICU stay began more than a month earlier. I took this as a *very* good sign – an alert mind is one of the most important factors in success after extubation, and it's rare to be able to crack a smile if you're hanging onto life by a thread.

Prayer 115 (July 19, 2020)
Lord – let my heart seek the things that are above, where Christ is, not the things of Earth. Hide me with Christ in God.
Put to death that which is earthly within me and give me life in Christ.
Fill me with compassion, kindness, humility, meekness and patience.
Help me forgive, as I have been forgiven by you Lord.
Let love and the peace of Christ rule in my heart – let his word dwell in me richly, teaching me wisdom.
Whatever I do, in word or deed, let it be in the name of the Lord Jesus, giving thanks and praise to God the Father through him.
[Derived from Colossians 3]

Lynn (*one of my many favorite nurses*) came down with Covid pneumonia, likely due to workplace exposure since she had been doing nothing but ICU shifts all month and her husband and daughter hadn't been ill. Lynn experienced high fevers, severe weakness and shortness of breath. She tested negative for Covid at work but retested *positive* a day later at a community testing site. After seeing what was going on in the hospital, she decided she didn't want to be admitted unless absolutely necessary. "You know, it was not looking good if you got admitted!" Her husband bought her an oximeter at Walgreens (a $40 device that clips over your fingertip and measures your O2 sat) and Lynn "self-proned" laying on her stomach whenever her O2 sat fell below 90%.

She decided (with uncustomary risk-taking) that she would report to the ER only if her O2 sat fell below 82%, rather than the standard threshold below 92% [*Two parenthetical comments: 1) Do as nurses and doctors say, not as they do, and 2) Lynn is a professional, do not try this at home!*]

On the tenth day of her illness, Lynn's O2 sat fell to 83% despite self-proning; she took a few puffs off an old asthma inhaler from her medicine cabinet and her O2 sats inched back up into the high 80s*. The next day, her fever broke and she began recovering. It took Lynn five weeks to return to work. [*Asthma inhalers provide no benefit for most people experiencing Covid pneumonia, but Covid can provoke asthma – perhaps that's why Lynn felt better after using her inhaler.*]

Prayer 116 (July 20, 2020)
Father, I come into your house and lay Christ's offering before you.
I will fulfill the vows my mouth promised when I was in trouble.
I offer to you Christ's sacrifice.
Come and hear, all who fear God and I will tell you what he's done for me!
Truly God has heard my cry and has not rejected my prayer or removed his steadfast love from me. Blessed be God Almighty!
[A modern version of Psalm 66]

Samuel, a 67-year-old man with Covid pneumonia, was almost three weeks into his ICU stay, proned, on 100% oxygen and maximal ventilator pressures. This morning, he suddenly went into rapid atrial fibrillation, and his blood pressure plummeted. As we supined him to shock him, he coded!

Mayfield was running codes that day, but Samuel was my patient, so we worked the code in tandem. After 15 minutes of CPR and three doses of intravenous epinephrine, we weren't getting anywhere. The echo machine arrived, and some quick ultrasound images of Samuel's chest revealed that *both* his lungs were ruptured! While Mayfield continued running the code, I emergently placed chest tubes to reinflate both his lungs while CPR was ongoing – first the left, then the right. I have to say; it was not the calm, controlled situation surgery should be.

We achieved "ROSC" – return of spontaneous circulation – soon thereafter. It took fifty minutes from the time Samuel coded to stabilize his condition enough to step away from his bedside. Mayfield and I took off our steaming-hot PPE outside the room. My scrub top underneath was as wet as if I had just been swimming in it – I must have sweated a gallon under the sterile surgical gown I was wearing. A tough code takes a lot out of you – adrenaline floods your bloodstream at first, but then it really bottoms out when you're done. Suddenly, I felt like I could sleep a hundred years if I could just lay my head down – *but I still had eight more hours to go this shift.*

A nurse kindly offered to help me reach Samuel's wife to let her know what happened, but we had trouble reaching her. About an hour later, we learned that Samuel's wife wasn't picking up her cell phone because she had turned it off for her daughter's funeral, who had died from Covid pneumonia earlier that week.

Prayer 117 (July 21, 2020)
Then the spirit of the Lord lifted me up and brought me to the gate of the house of the Lord . . .
You said, "I will execute my judgment upon you, and you will know I am Lord."
I fell facedown and cried out in a loud voice, "Alas Lord, will you completely destroy the remnant of your people on Earth?"

Lord, gather your scattered people and bring us together with one heart and be our sanctuary.
Open our eyes to see you. Open our ears to hear you.
Put a new spirit in us.
Remove our hearts of stone and give us hearts of flesh, so that we

may walk in your ways, and we shall be your people forever.
[Inspired by Ezekiel 11 and 12]

The number of Covid deaths in Arizona (and in many other locations around the world) overcame the ability of funeral homes to bury or cremate the bodies. The capacity of our hospital morgue ("four bodies, maybe six if we played Tetris," according to one of our security team) was quickly overwhelmed and hospital administration decided to acquire a refrigerated truck in which dead bodies could be stored in the parking lot out behind the hospital. They did not initially appreciate that the refrigeration unit ran off the gas engine, so the truck had to idle 24 hours per day. This created a potentially macabre job for the security guards, who thought at first they might have to periodically drive the truck full of dead bodies to the gas station to "fill-er up." But this didn't come to pass as a company that could deliver gasoline to the vehicle was engaged.

Prayer 118 (July 22, 2020)
Blessed be the God and Father of our Lord Jesus Christ, who has blessed us in Christ with every spiritual blessing.
In him we have redemption through his blood, the forgiveness of our trespasses according to the riches of his grace, which he lavished upon us in all wisdom and insight.
He made known to us the mystery of his will according to his purpose, which he set forth in Christ as a plan for the fullness of time, to unite all things in him, things in Heaven and things on Earth. [From Ephesians 1]

As we continued to wean Clayton off sedation, he finally began interacting and we discovered that he couldn't move his left arm or leg. He was completely neglecting the left half of his body as if it didn't exist anymore. A CT of his brain showed he had suffered two strokes on the right side of his brain, most likely a few days previously. We had no way of knowing exactly when they occurred because the heavy sedation he required had completely obscured his neurological findings over the preceding weeks.

Prayer 119 (July 23, 2020)

The universe is your handiwork Lord, proclaiming your glory!
You have set the sun in the Heavens and marked out its path across the sky.
No wonder, the fear of the Lord will endure forever!
Your law warns your servant, your commandments open our eyes, and your mercy washes our souls clean.
Declare me innocent from fault.
Keep back your servant from evil – let it not have dominion over me! Then I shall be blameless in your sight.
I pray that the words of my mouth and the meditation of my heart be acceptable in your sight, O Lord, my rock and my redeemer!
[Psalm 19 abbreviated again – I sure love this one!]

July 2020. The Southern sky as seen from Payson Arizona just after moonrise.

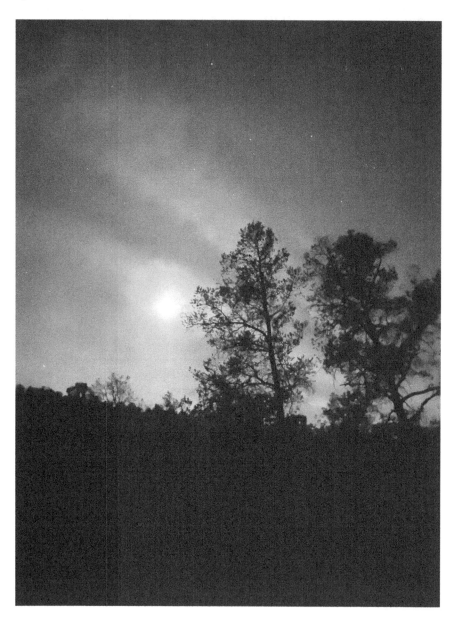

"The Heavens declare the glory of God." There is a type of neutron star called a "Magnetar" which has a mass many times that of our sun. It is so compacted that a teaspoon weighs 100 million tons. The magnetic field of a magnetar is so strong that you would die if you approached within 1000 kilometers, as it stripped all the electrons of your atoms. If you somehow stood on the surface of a magnetar, the gravitational gradient would be so enormous that it would pull your body apart in a process aptly (and to my nerdish delight) called "spaghettification."

Yet, quasars are far, *far* more powerful than magnetars. They are super-massive black holes that weigh a billion times more than our sun and consume the equivalent of 10 times the mass of the Earth per second, producing up to 1000 times more
energy than the entire Milky Way galaxy – 10,000,000,000,000,000,000,000,000,000,000,000,000,000 watts of energy. They are the most luminous objects in the known universe, visible to our telescopes at a distance of over 29 billion light-years. Some quasars produce titanic X-ray jets that extend a million light-years into space.

Our God made these things. He commands them – objects that would annihilate our entire solar system on an atomic level if we even remotely entered their cosmic proximity. Yet, *their* Master invites us safely into his presence through the sacrifice of his Son.

Prayer 120 (July 24, 2020)
You did not require a sacrifice from me to come before you, thanks to your Son, I only had to call the name Jesus.
Here I am – I have come before you poor and needy.
I have nothing to offer but my desire to do your will my God.
Put your law in my heart.
I will not deny your mighty works.
I will not conceal your loving-kindness.

But I will shout your praises from the rooftops!
Do not withhold your mercy from me Lord.
May your love and faithfulness always protect me.
For troubles without number surround me –
I am drowning in a sea of adversity and my heart is failing within
me. Do not forsake me Lord – come quickly!
You are my mighty Lord and deliverer.
[Another interpretation of Psalm 40]

On July 24, 2020, 89 people died from Covid in Arizona – the highest daily Covid death toll recorded that summer.

The previously healthy 48-year-old Clayton was transferred to a nursing home, a shell of his former self. Trached and PEGed (having had a Percutaneous Endoscopic Gastrostomy feeding tube surgically placed through the wall of his stomach), still on a vent, receiving dialysis, diabetic, his left side paralyzed from two strokes and barely able to sit on the side of the bed without assistance, after 35 days in the hospital. He was one of the "lucky Covid survivors."

Prayer 121 (July 26, 2020)
My strength, my salvation, my very life comes from the mighty Creator of Heaven and Earth.
The God of Israel and his Son Jesus.
He who never sleeps, he who is never surprised by anything that befalls me, or anything I do.
He who always forgives, no matter how often and awfully I fail.
He always counts me as he would his beloved Son.
The Lord is my shade during the heat of day and my shelter in the cold night. He watches over my coming and going both now and forevermore, protecting me from all harm.
In his grace, I cannot fail. [Another interpretation of Psalm 121]

As our patient census plateaued at new record highs, I became an automaton at work, focused completely on getting all my work done as efficiently as possible. You don't realize how much time you "waste" each workday until you are under this sort of pressure. I became entirely task-driven from the minute I walked through the hospital door. Samantha grabbed my elbow, wanting to share a funny story, but I told her I didn't have time. As I walked down the halls from one patient room to another, I constantly pushed my walking pace faster. I mentally scheduled when I could go to the bathroom depending on the immediacy of the patient care tasks on my list each given moment.

Prayer 122 (July 28, 2020)
Lord, creator of the universe, yet loving Father to a bunch of pipsqueak old guys* on a minuscule world.
How do you operate on such hugely different scales?
We praise you and thank you for a few of your inventions:
Thanks for life, the beautiful world you made us, the promise of rain.
Thanks for restful sleep last night and being physically able to do what we need to do today.
Thanks for all the good people keeping our world running – the grocery clerks and car repairmen and nurses.
Thanks for 70's music and jokes.
Thanks for the good food we ate today, for our clothes and our houses, a glass of wine and putting our feet up after work.
Thanks for our wives and kids.
Thanks for honesty, courtesy and kind intentions.
Thanks for the Bible, for your mercy and grace.
Thanks for faith and thanks for love. What a great day!
[*referring to me and my bible-study brothers*]

Vincenzo was discharged to rehab. We didn't find out what happened to him there until almost two months later.

Prayer 123 (July 31, 2020)
We thank you for your church, founded upon your word, that challenges us to do more than sing and pray, but go out and work as though the very answer to our prayers depended on us and not upon you.

Help us to realize that humanity was created to shine like the stars and live on through all eternity.
Keep us, we pray, in perfect peace.
Help us to walk together, pray together, sing together, and live together until that day when all God's children – Black, White, Red, Brown and Yellow – will rejoice in one common band of humanity in the reign of our Lord and of our God,
we pray. Amen. [Dr. Martin King Jr.]

Samuel, the patient who needed two chest tubes to survive his code, went on to slowly recover over the next few weeks and eventually came off the ventilator. Samuel was transferred to a long-term care facility after 38 days in the ICU. We were incredulous to learn shortly thereafter that he died less than 24 hours later. All the pain he suffered, all our work, culminating only in a brief and false recovery – all for nothing. The only good thing left is that Samuel died without learning about the death of his son.

Prayer 124 (August 2, 2020)
My soul boasts in the Lord; let the humble hear and be glad.
Oh magnify the Lord with me and let us exalt his name together!
I sought the Lord and he answered me
and delivered me from all my fears.
This poor man cried out, and the Lord heard!

Oh taste and see that the Lord is good!
Blessed is the man who takes refuge in him.
The eyes of the Lord are toward the righteous and his ears hear their cry.
The Lord is near to the brokenhearted and saves the crushed in spirit.
Many are the afflictions of the righteous, but the Lord delivers him out of them all.
None who take refuge in him will be forsaken.
[Psalm 34 abbreviated]

I had been missing our Friday 6 am Bible study because I

worked most Fridays; the early morning was prime time to get on top of the day's work. I texted the group: "I'm really sorry I missed the discussion on forgiveness in Bible study the other day. I read the same passages you guys did. I know the actions I need to take and why I need to take them, but I can't change my heart by any effort of my own will. I can't think of this *one guy*, who ended my prior career, without hating him."

I received this reply: "Ask Jesus to accomplish the forgiveness in you. I couldn't do it on my own, either. It had to be done by Jesus. Just ask and believe he can move any mountain."

Prayer 125 (August 5, 2020)
Lord, your holy Son pointed out to us that you are kind even to the ungrateful and the wicked.
And that we are not to judge or condemn or demand repayment from each other for wrongs visited upon us.

In obedience, I pray for this man I hate.
Please bless him, his wife and family.
Please have mercy on him for his mistakes and forgive him.
Give him wisdom not to repeat them.
In my book, from this point forward, he doesn't owe me anything.
If I ever meet him again and have a chance, let me do him a kindness.

But Lord – only you can fix my heart! I tried and failed many times. Please lift this burden of shame and anger from me for once and all Lord and free me from hating this man. I ask this in the name of your Son, Jesus.

I had been employed by a large teaching hospital for 34 years before leaving for my current job in 2018. During that long tenure, Novak and I established a sustainable system for providing the best care we could for our ICU patients without focusing on money. But that all changed in 2014, under new management, and after a prolonged conflict, I felt compelled to quit my job, leaving behind beloved colleagues and a practice that I had helped build over decades. I frequently thought of the administrator who was the source of that conflict when I said the Lord's prayer, because I had never been able to sincerely forgive him, and I couldn't bring myself to say, "Forgive us our trespasses as we forgive those who trespass against us" so long as my hate endured. (You may have noticed this in previous versions of the Lord's prayer I have shared). I don't know what made me think of him more than two years later, but I found today that I could pray for him as Jesus commanded.

"As for you, you meant evil against me, but God meant it for good" [Genesis 50:20]. If I hadn't been pushed out of my old job, I wouldn't have gotten to work with Mayfield, Joyce, and the entire team here in our ICU. I knew I was right where God wanted me to be.

Prayer 126 (August 8, 2020)
Lord, whether we are in dire straights, or we think we are sailing along, it is only by your loving-kindness that we will survive today.
We have complete faith that you can tell Estelle "Get up and walk out of the hospital" and she will walk out of here one day.
Please let that be your will Lord. Heal her, body and mind.
Bless and protect her children, her family.
We dare to ask all blessings in the name of your holy Son Jesus – the saver of our souls!

We had been experiencing an extraordinarily high rate of barotrauma in our Covid pneumonia patients. Barotrauma is the technical term used when the lung ruptures from pneumonia (or a number of other processes) and the pressure generated by the ventilator forces air out through the leaking lung into the mediastinum (the core of the chest between the lungs) and from there, up under the skin of the neck, head and chest. Sometimes this pressurized air collects inside the chest cavity collapsing the adjacent lung. The resulting "pneumothorax" can be fatal if not evacuated in time.

Estelle was an intubated 64-year-old woman with Covid pneumonia experiencing severe barotrauma. Her face, neck and chest were grossly distorted by the pressurized air dissecting under her skin. Her eyelids were swollen shut, stretched to translucency; her head looked like a melon. She had already experienced a pneumothorax of the left lung and I was anticipating the right lung could go any time. We had turned her ventilator pressures down as much as we could, but it was a "Catch-22" – she needed high ventilator pressures to force oxygen into her ravaged lungs.

That afternoon, our most experienced nurse, Pam, paged me urgently that Estelle's O2 sats and blood pressure had suddenly plummeted. The first we both thought was that Estelle had developed a pneumothorax on the right.

I arrived with the ultrasound machine in tow and scanned the right lung. It was down – pneumothorax! I looked up at the Philips ICU monitor: O2 sat at 84%, heart rate 108, blood pressure 91/58. *Borderline – I better hurry.* "Pam – crank her up to 100% oxygen."

I knew exactly where all the equipment I needed to place a chest tube was stored and I could fetch it myself quicker than asking someone else to find it. I asked Pam to give 50 micrograms of fentanyl to help Estelle tolerate the procedure – *hopefully without dropping her blood pressure* – and ran off to grab the chest tube surgical kit, my sterile gown and gloves.

I was back in the room within a minute, pulled the drapes shut for some privacy, flattened out Estelle's bed, set up my kit on a bedside table and pulled the bedsheets and gown away to expose her chest. I quickly scrubbed the skin under Estelle's armpit with orange betadine solution, donned my surgical gown and gloves and looked up at the monitor: O2 sat 83%, heart rate 110, blood pressure 89/57. *Go, go, go!*

I covered Estelle's body with a bed-sized fenestrated sterile barrier – the fenestration was a round cut-out about 10cm in diameter that I centered over the area on Estelle's chest wall where I was going to operate, at the level of the fifth rib in mid-axillary line (below the middle of the armpit). Estelle's breast was in the field, and I asked Pam to reach under the sterile field and hold it out of the way. I injected lidocaine into the skin over the fifth rib, probing deeper until the needle struck the bone and emptying the syringe there. Then I made a deep nick in the anesthetized skin with a scalpel. I picked up a syringe and large-bore needle, directing the needle through the incision until I hit the rib, then inched the tip upwards and over the top of the rib – *the intercostal artery lay <u>under</u> the rib, and I definitely didn't want to puncture that.* The syringe filled with air as the needle entered the pleural space surrounding the ruptured lung. This is right where I wanted to be! I popped the syringe off the needle, careful not to let the needle position shift, then passed a steel guidewire through the needle and into the chest. Now the needle could be removed and a dilator passed over the wire to create a tract for insertion of the chest tube. The dilator was thicker than a Bic ballpoint pen, and took some pressure to pop it through the pleura over the guidewire. When I pulled the dilator out, a hiss of air exited Estelle's chest. This was some of the pressurized air collapsing Estelle's lung – a good sign that the guidewire was in the right place. I looked up at the monitor: O2 sat 81%, heart rate 115, blood pressure 82/52 – *things were beginning to fall apart, better speed up.* "Pam – hang some Levophed!" (a life-support drug that boosts blood pressure)

The chest tube itself was 40 cm and had an internal dilator to give it rigidity and help it pop through the pleura, but as I passed it over the guidewire, it seemed to get hung up on something between the ribs. I tried a few times from slightly different angles, rotating the chest tube over the wire and pushing a little harder, but it wouldn't pass into the chest. I pulled it out to examine it – the tip of the internal dilator was bent – this was the tip of the spear and the chest tube wasn't going anywhere unless that dilator tip went there first. Monitor: O2 sat 79%, heart rate 118, blood pressure 84/63. *Come on, come on!*

I tried to fix the damaged silastic dilator tip with my fingernail and passed the assembly over the guidewire again. It hung up again. I wasn't getting anywhere. I would never successfully place the chest tube if the guidewire was also bent, but the only way to tell was to pull the guidewire out and that meant virtually starting the procedure all over. Monitor: O2 sat 77%, heart rate 121, blood pressure 79/55. *Lord, help!* I pulled the wire out – it was badly kinked! Useless. I tossed it off the sterile field.

"Pam– I need another chest tube kit right away, please!" Pam scooted off – the procedure kits were stocked nearby and within a minute, she returned and handed me a new sterile procedure kit.

Monitor: O2 sat 75%, heart rate 82, blood pressure 72/52. Moving as fast as I could, I repeated the insertion technique, exerting some extra effort with dilation. This time the chest tube passed about 25 cm into the pleural space with ease.

Monitor: O2 sat 69%, heart rate 48, blood pressure 68/42. Estelle was "bradying down" – *her heart rate plummeting, heralding impending respiratory arrest.* I connected the chest tube to the pleural evacuation container and Pam turned the suction on full; gas began vigorously bubbling out of Estelle's chest into the container. *Success!*

Monitor: O2 sat at 85%, heart rate 75, blood pressure 85/52 and rising. The bed was a wreck – *I was a wreck.* Pam was unperturbed, as though nothing out of the ordinary had happened. That chest tube placement should have gone smoothly, but it nearly cost Estelle her life. Thank God she hung in there long enough for me to finally complete the job.

Prayer 127 (August 9, 2020)
O God, you are my God.
My soul thirsts for you in a dry and weary land where there is no water.
In my bed, I think of you through the watches of the night.
I sing in the shadows of your wings.

My soul clings to you, your right hand upholds me.
I will praise you as long as I live. [Psalm 63 abbreviated]

Pam was a wonder. She had been an ICU nurse for most of her 45-year career and somehow also raised eight kids! Now in her seventies, she was unflappable, having "seen everything". She couldn't have been taller than 4'6" and looked like she weighed 80 lbs. soaking wet, but she had the supernatural physical strength all good nurses seem to possess. She told me she had no intention of ever retiring, planned on "working 'til the day I die – why shouldn't I? I still love it." I tried vainly to get Pam's goat, employing a variety of knick-names for her, including "Short-timer" and "Rookie." She never paid me any attention. She never showed any annoyance, but neither would she smile or laugh at my foolishness.

I noted that many of the world's best people go into ICU nursing, but few last very long. Some shake out quickly. Others work 5-10 years before moving on to other areas of the hospital – the post-op recovery unit, maybe dialysis. A few – *in my experience, almost exclusively women* – stay in the ICU for 15-25 years or more. These are the heart of the nursing unit, who seem to know what to do in any emergency I worry their experience and mentoring of the younger nurses is sometimes under-appreciated by administrators who have never worked side by side with them. If a senior bedside nurse left our unit for any reason, she could not be replaced. Finally, there was Pam – who stood alone on top of the longevity pyramid. She had smartly withdrawn a little from jumping feet first into every emergency, but she could still hold her own, as she aptly demonstrated.

Prayer 128 (August 10, 2020)
God, we thank you for the inspiration of Jesus.
Grant that we will love you with all our hearts, souls, and minds, and love our neighbors as we love ourselves, even our enemy neighbors.

And we ask you, God, in these days of emotional tension, when the problems of the world are gigantic in extent and chaotic in detail, to be with us in our going out and our coming in, in our rising up and in our lying down, in our moments of joy and in our moments of sorrow, until the day when there shall be no sunset and no dawn. Amen

[Dr. Martin Luther King Jr.]

One of my old ICU partners back in the days I worked with Dom – Dr. Jan O'Neil – reached out to see how I was doing and commiserate. Jan worked the ICU night shift all her career, taking care of her husband and two children during the day. *I never figured out when she slept.* Of all the physicians I helped train and work with over the years, Jan was my favorite and the one whose opinion meant the most to me, especially now that Dom was gone. Jan was at the peak of her career, soon to be Chief of Staff at the hospital where she worked, but her heart was still in the right place. We were on the phone sharing some theories about optimal ventilator settings for Covid patients when Jan confided in me she felt much of the humanity had gone out of our jobs. So many of the patients were uncommunicative due to BiPAP masks or intubation – their families were restricted from visiting. It was becoming hard to remember that these were human beings in the ICU beds. Jan confirmed what I had been feeling, but neither of us had an any easy solution.

Prayer 129 (August 12, 2020)
Praise awaits you, our God, to you our vows will be fulfilled.
You who answer prayer, to you all people will come.
When we were overwhelmed by sins, you forgave our transgressions.
Blessed are those you choose and bring near to live in your courts!
We are filled with the good things of your house, of your holy temple.
God our Savior, the hope of all the ends of the Earth and of the farthest seas, who formed the mountains by your power, who

stilled the roaring of the seas; the whole Earth is filled with awe at your wonders.
[from Psalm 65, part 1]

Prayer 130 (August 14, 2020)
Where morning dawns, where evening fades, you call forth songs of joy.
You care for the land and water.
The streams of God are filled with water to provide the people with grain, for so you have ordained.
You soften the Earth with showers and bless its crops.
You crown the year with your bounty.
The grasslands of the wilderness overflow; the hills are clothed with gladness.
The meadows are covered with flocks and the valleys mantled with grain. They shout for joy and sing praises to your name.
[Psalm 65 part 2]

August 20, 2020. *Sunrise behind the McDowell Mountains, 5:30am.*

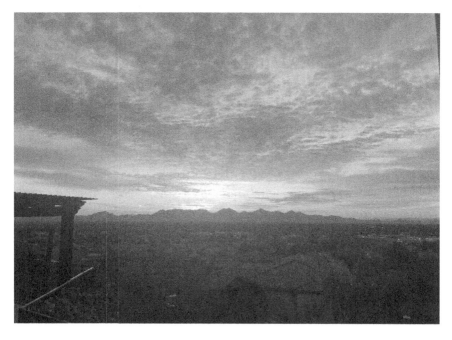

Prayer 131 (August 21, 2020)

Almighty God – heavenly Father, who feeds and clothes all creation – deliver me, in my work, from falling into the temptation of putting reputation or money in the forefront.
Help me perform the job you've given me for the benefit of my brothers and sisters, in the name of your Son Jesus Christ, who lived and died to serve us – the undeserving.
Lord – let my heart seek the things that are above, where Christ is, not the things of Earth.
Hide me with Christ in God.
Put to death that which is earthly within me and give me life in Christ.
Fill me with compassion, kindness, humility and patience.
Help me forgive, as I have been forgiven by you Lord.
Let love and the peace of Christ rule in my heart – let his Word dwell in me richly, teaching me wisdom.
Whatever I do, in word or deed, let it be in the name of the Lord Jesus, giving thanks and praise to God the Father through him.
[Derived from Colossians 3:1-17]

I came up with an idea pursuant to my discussion with my old partner Jan: to speak out loud to each patient, even if they were comatose; to *physically touch* each patient (maybe on their brow, their shoulder), and most importantly, to pray aloud for each patient at their bedside every day. Among other things, this gave me a renewed reason to enter the rooms of proned patients.

I had been trying this out for about a week with some recovery of my sense of humanity when I asked our hospital chaplain what he thought of the idea. I had an inkling he might be excited and might even organize a system of prayer rounds with patients whose families OKed it. But his response surprised me.

"What if they don't want to be prayed for? You don't have the right to pray for them without their consent." I clammed up – realizing I had perhaps been unwise to share my excitement. I had never been restrained from praying with patients at the hospital, and I wanted to keep it that way.

I was a bit discouraged, but I knew I couldn't stop now. In my experience, most patients want to be prayed for, *or are at least OK with it.* Only a few times through the years has a patient flatly refused a prayer offer. Now, without family visitation, the patients were more alone than ever before. I felt strongly that praying for them was a way of letting them know they were not alone, that someone cared about them as a person. And it wasn't only for the patients' benefit – *I desperately needed to do this.* Praying in each room was rekindling humanity to the conduct of my work. It might be the only thing that could keep me going.

I secretly made one concession to the chaplain: I started asking families for prayer consent when I called to report to them. In most cases, prayer had already been going on for a number of days by this point, *but better to ask for forgiveness than permission.* In cases where I couldn't obtain family permission, I prefaced each prayer with "I hope you don't mind if I pray for you."

Prayer 132 (August 23, 2020)
I cry out to the Lord; I plead for mercy.
I tell my troubles before him.
When my spirit fails within me, you know my way!
On the path I walk, there are traps hidden for me – no refuge remains but you.
I cry out to you, "You are my refuge – my portion in the land of the living."
Deliver me from evil – it is too strong for me!
Bring me out of prison, so that I can give thanks to your name!
Your righteousness will surround me and you will pour out your blessings upon me!
[Derived from Psalm 142, a prayer of David when he resided in a cave.]

Several times, events unfolded that made me falsely (and megalomaniacally) believe I had made a breakthrough in the treatment of Covid. But every time a new technique seemed to work, it turned out to be a fluke. One such case involved a patient named Sanford, who had been mechanically ventilated and proned for 22 days when I picked up his care. We had previously established a protocol for getting patients out of proning beds; this was a crucial first step in recovery since once proning was discontinued, sedation could be dropped and the ventilator weaned as the patient awoke. The protocol involved comparing O2 sats in proned and supined positions each day – when they were approximately equal, the benefit of proning had been exhausted and the patient could be supined. Sanford was making absolutely no progress on this protocol; his O2 sat was consistently better proned every day for the past three weeks. This wasn't getting him anywhere. I decided Sanford's best chance was to forget about our protocol.

Prayer 133 (August 24, 2020)
Sanford – I hope you don't mind me praying for you.
Don't you give up brother. Keep fighting.
I pray for you to our Father God in Heaven.
I have no authority to do so, but our savior Jesus the Son has all authority, in Heaven and on Earth.
I pray through him to the Father to heal you.
And if Jesus will just smile your way, just his slightest nod yes, you will be healed.
Our medicines don't work unless he says so.
Lord just say the word – heal Sanford today.

I supined Sanford and kept him face-up. His O2 sats fell but not dangerously. I had the nurses remove the proning bed from his room for use by another patient to eliminate reproning temptation (like Cortez burning his boats). Over the next five days, I relentlessly lowered Sanford's ventilator settings and sedation drug dosages, regardless of whether it appeared that he could tolerate it. It worked like magic. By the end of my block of shifts, Sanford's oxygen requirement had fallen from 100% to 40%, and he was awake enough to extubate. I thought I was a genius until I tried it on several other of our patients. The part where I just turned the ventilator settings down each day never worked again. Still, it helped Sanford get out of the ICU, and among those as sick as Sanford, every success was worth celebrating.

Prayer 134 (August 25, 2020)
There is none like you, O Lord, nor are there any works like yours.
All nations shall one day come and worship before you, and shall glorify your name. You alone are God!

Hear me Lord and answer me, for I am sorely in need.
You are my God; have mercy on me.
I call to you all day long, for you answer me.
Bring help to your servant Lord, for I put my trust in you.
You are a compassionate and gracious God, slow to anger, abounding in love and faithfulness.
Turn to me and have mercy on me; show your strength in behalf of your servant. For great is your love toward me; you have delivered me from the depths, even from the realm of the dead.
[Derived from Psalm 86]

Prayer 135 (August 27, 2020)
God and Father of all, whom the Heavens adore, let the Earth also worship you, all nations obey you, all tongues confess and praise you, all men and women everywhere love you and serve you in peace through Jesus Christ our Lord.
Inspire me to encourage others by what I say and do.
Never let me look down on my brother, but show me how to love as Christ did, in his holy name and for your glory.

One of our Covid patients, an 80-year-old named Vera, was slowly deteriorating despite our highest level of life support. She was unconscious for the entirety of her 24-day ICU admission, and had never really interacted except to grimace and withdraw her limbs weakly when I applied painful pressure to her fingernails and toenails each day – *a regrettable necessity of our daily neurological exam for which I repeatedly apologized.* Her skin was pale and swollen from all the IV fluids she had received – translucent as gelatin. The tissues of her neck and upper chest were full of gas. You could feel it with your fingertips, even through the gloves – *what we call "crepitus"* – the gentle subcutaneous popping of air bubbles that have leaked out of rupturing lungs and spread under the skin. I had lost hope for Vera over the course of the last few days. I had to call her husband Heck:

"Heck, it's Dr. Eckshar. I'm calling about Vera."

"How is she a doctor? Is she getting any better?"

"I'm sorry, Heck. Vera is *not* getting any better. I wish I didn't have to tell you this, but Vera is not *going* to get any better. Her lungs just won't heal. I don't think she can go on like this much longer."

"Doc, is there *any* chance at all?"

Of course, there was almost always some miniscule chance – one in a thousand? It's possible ongoing life support could artificially draw out Vera's death process for weeks – but would she ever go home? Chat with Heck in the kitchen while making dinner together? Bounce her grandkids on her knee? – I thought not. I had to internally acknowledge some uncertainty, but Heck needed certainty from me for his conscience to be clear, so I gave it to him.

"No Heck, there is no chance at all."

"I know. I guess I've known that for some time. Are you saying I gotta let her go?" his deep voice cracked.

"I think it's time, Heck."

"I understand, Doc. You know, Vera hasn't seen a doctor in 40 years – since she had the kids – no, that's 45 years now." He chuckled a little, "Sorry doc, but she didn't like you doctor-types very much. She did her *own* doctoring – for herself and the kids when they were little." Then plaintively, "If we turn the machines off . . . can't I come see her?" *He knew the rules – knew there was no visiting a Covid patient under any circumstances – even these.*

"No, Heck. I really wish you could – *I truly meant that* – but we can't let any visitors come up here to our Covid ward. It's not safe."

Resigned: "OK. When are we going to do this?"

"Whenever you're ready." I explained the process to Heck – how we would give Vera some morphine and Versed (an anxiety–relieving drug akin to valium) and then extubate her and let her breathe naturally. Sam and I would give more meds generously for any sign that Vera was suffering. Heck agreed, and I called together Sam and June and told them the plan. Shortly, they had everything ready and I called Heck back. "I'm holding my cell phone up to her ear now. Heck – we're taking Vera off the vent now – you can say goodbye to her."

"Ver – honey – it's Heck. I wish I could be there with you, honey, hold your hand again, give you a kiss – but they won't let me. They won't let me honey. I love you Ver . . . 57 years. We took good care of each other for 57 years, didn't we? – rain or shine. You're a good wife, Ver, the best, and I love you. You are the only one for me, the only one I will ever love." He stumbled, "I don't know what else to say . . . You go ahead now, Ver, go ahead, honey. Don't worry about me. You just rest now. I love you."

It wasn't right, my being party to these last words between a husband and wife. But I was blessed by it. When I walked into Vera's room that morning, it was hard to see Vera as anything more than a decrepit octogenarian on her deathbed, a name to cross off my over-flowing worklist after she died. Now, she was the love of Heck's life.

At least Heck was blameless. But I knew someday I would stand before God and find out whether I acted according to his will or not in this matter.

Prayer 136 (August 30, 2020)
Prayer in the room of a comatose patient:
Lord, bless Jorge (I laid my gloved hand on his brow).

Bless his family.
Get him through today with no pain, no setbacks, no fear –
Lord, let him know you are with him and you are in charge.
No harm can befall him under your protection.
Nothing is beyond you –

Just say the word Lord and Jorge will be healed.
You can do it in an instant if you want Lord.
We know we might have to wait for healing in your time but please
hurry.
Say the word and Jorge will breath on his own again.
Let him recover quickly now Lord and get him home with his family
and friends. In your holy name we pray.

Jorge was a feeble 79-year-old gentleman who looked like he would die from Covid pneumonia from the get-go. He arrived intubated, so I never got the chance to talk with him. If his family could have visited, they might have posted pictures in his room of Jorge in shorts and a T-shirt out fishing on Apache Lake and pictures of his twelve grandkids opening presents on Christmas. They might have told us he was a Vietnam War veteran, a gourmet chef, or that he had traveled to over 100 foreign countries (as one dying patient's family once told me). But Jorge's family couldn't visit, and I didn't know one personal thing about Jorge.

When we interrupted Jorge's sedation drugs, he awoke unable to talk or move (being intubated and in soft restraints), disoriented, possibly delirious and surrounded by masked strangers. [*A patient who survived two weeks of mechanical ventilation for severe influenza pneumonia once told me she thought she was in a Nazi crematorium.*] So, it's not surprising that Jorge almost immediately required the resumption of heavy sedation. How different that might be if only Jorge could awaken to see his wife, his son, holding his hands, whispering to him it was going to be OK.

I applauded the restriction of family visitation as an infection control procedure back in March 2020. It took me six months to fully realize what we had sacrificed – what the families had sacrificed. I finally realized what a mistake we had made. *We needed the families back.*

Prayer 137 (September 1, 2020)
Saw this majestic elk calmly foraging at dusk yesterday in Payson. He reminded me of God's quiet dominion on Earth – immune to our mistakes – speaking quietly to those who have ears – offering peace and protection to those who ask it of him.

September 1, 2020. *A bull elk grazing off the side of the road, Payson AZ*

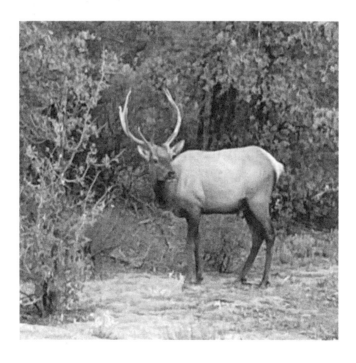

The natural world God created had become a great source of peace for us, *perhaps some primordial memory of how life had been in the garden of Eden.*

Jean and I were taking a walk down the street on the edge

of town around sunset when we came across this beautiful elk grazing on the ground cover by the side of the road. We approached silently, respectfully, as near as we dared, and froze there watching him. He took only momentary notice of us, then calmly went back to foraging. I thought about all the things going on in our world that were so out of control, so frightening – and how they didn't matter at all to this elk. He was a creature under God's protection. The natural world would go on.

Prayer 138 (September 2, 2020)
God, you so loved the world that you sent your only Son so that whoever believes in him should not perish but have eternal life.
You did not send your Son into the world to condemn the world, but in order that the world might be saved through him.
Your light came into this world, yet so many loved the darkness instead of the light.
For them we pray. Lord, enlarge your flock.
Pour your grace down again on the undeserving, as you did for us.
Grant them faith. Open their eyes to your omnipresence in the world around us, so they can see your loving hand and your purpose in all that happens.
Forgive their sins and bless them Lord, as you have blessed us.
And let us be part of your work for their salvation.
We love you and trust you Lord. [Based on John 3]

Over the course of the next several months, I asked every conscious patient whether they were OK with me praying for them. All of them said yes and most were clearly grateful. In relation to unconscious patients, I asked permission from every family that I spoke to, and all granted it. A few seemed semi-amused – *perhaps they agreed only to humor me* – but most were sincerely appreciative.

I put my gloved hand on Jorge's brow and prayed for him again today, as I had been doing every day. A tear rolled down his cheek – perhaps the only means of communication left to him. I don't know exactly what that tear meant – *appreciation of human touch, of hope? Maybe the tears of a prodigal son returning to the loving arms of his heavenly Father?* In any case, at least I felt I did some good coming into Jorge's room that day.

Prayer 139 (September 3, 2020)
Our God is the one and only, and his Son is always with him, interceding for those who the Father gave him, those that believe.
Our God is holy and all-powerful.
Our God listens to the prayers of his children and has mercy.
Our God loved us so much, he died on a cross to reconcile our sins.
Our God works fantastic, unimaginable miracles, healing all those who come to him.
All thanks and all praise and all glory to our God – Father, Son and Holy Spirit.
He has filled our hearts with hope and faith.

Prayer 140 (September 4, 2020)
Father, the hour has come: glorify your Son, so that your Son can glorify you!
You have given him authority to give eternal life to all whom you have given to him.
And this is eternal life: that we will know you, the only true God, and your son, Jesus Christ, whom you sent to save us.
Jesus glorified you on Earth, accomplishing all you gave him to do, and now Father, you glorify Jesus in your heavenly presence with all the glory he had with you before the world existed.
[The High Priestly prayer of Jesus, John 17, part 1]

I was starting a block of shifts Friday after having been off-duty for five days. One of our palliative care specialists sought me out early in the morning to inform me one of our patients was scheduled to transition to comfort care. Terrence was a 68-year-old Native American who had been in the ICU for four weeks with Covid pneumonia, showing no signs of recovery. He was in a coma, making no progress weaning from the vent, and required two pressors to maintain his blood pressure. The family had agreed to withdraw life support at 10 o'clock this morning. Seventeen family members had FaceTimed with him overnight to say their goodbyes.

I had not been involved with this difficult decision but was now responsible for carrying it through. Mayfield had warned me this was coming and recommended I look at the decision closely – *something about it must have been bothering him*. I reviewed the chart carefully. Terrence's chest X-ray was somewhat improved, and he was only receiving 40% oxygen (most of our really sick Covid pneumonia patients required 60–100% oxygen to maintain their O2 sats). Terrence was on six different sedation and analgesic drugs, each added for his comfort along the course of his ICU stay. Laying in a bed for a month on a ventilator is no doubt a terrible experience and none of us wanted our patients to suffer, but patients have to emerge from sedation to have any chance to get off the vent. Terrence's sedation meds hadn't been interrupted in several days.

Palliative care didn't entirely approve of my upsetting the applecart, but agreed when I asked them to give me a little time to be sure we were doing the right thing. I called Terrence's daughter, apologized for prolonging this difficult process and requested that she allow me over the weekend to give Terrence one more chance. She agreed without hesitation – *they weren't really very eager to give-in to Covid*. She mentioned that their family believed in traditional medicine, so I just said my own silent prayer that God would bless the course I was taking. I didn't want to torture Terrence, but we didn't have much time, so I completely discontinued all sedative and analgesic medications rather than gradually reducing them. I waited with anticipation to see what would happen next.

Prayer 141 (September 5, 2020)
We were made by you Father, chosen by you, and given to your Son, and your son gave us your word.
We know that Jesus came from you and that he's in Heaven with

you now.
But while we are stuck here on Earth, keep us in your name.
We know your Son is interceding on our behalf.
Let us be one with him and with you, heavenly Father.
Let us have Christ's joy fulfilled in our hearts.
We are not of this world anymore on account of your grace.
Jesus has sent us out the same way you sent him out – strangers in a strange land – hated by the world. Sanctify us in your truth.
[Adaption of the High Priestly prayer of Christ, John 17, part 2]

By the time I arrived at work early Saturday morning, Terrence no longer required pressor blood pressure support (two of the sedation drugs he had been receiving had the side effect of lowering blood pressure).

By Sunday, Terrence was starting to grimace and withdraw to nailbed pressure. [*Coma is loosely defined as the inability to interact with your environment due to an unconscious state. When a patient's fingernails are pinched, and they grimace and pull their hand away, it's a sign that they can experience painful sensations, process them and take appropriate action – not fully awake, but no longer in a coma per se.*]

Prayer 142 (September 7, 2020)
I had a nightmare last night and couldn't get back asleep.
Got pissed at work about some trivial paperwork.
Came home to some troubles with our in-laws.
Never caught sight of what's important all day long.

Father, you created the universe, created us, in accordance with your plan for us. Jesus suffered and died for me.
Not for me to fuss over paperwork, but for me to enjoy life to its fullest, loving and serving like Jesus did, glorifying you on Earth in everything I think say and do.
Thank you for giving us a life of great purpose Lord.
But I would waste it all without your constant daily guidance.
Be my shepherd Lord. Guide me in right paths.
Free me from fear and let me dwell in your house forever!

On September 8th, Terrence was fully awake, able to obey requests such as "show me two fingers" and successfully extubated. He went on to transfer to rehab and recovered fully. We were getting near the end of the Summer 2020 Covid surge, and our attention was increasingly focused on getting patients like Terrence *off* the vents rather than putting them on.

A new Covid unit visitation policy was announced, but not what I had been hoping for. Families could now visit Covid patients in the unit wearing the proper PPE, *but only* if the patient was being transitioned to comfort care. Most such patients were expected to expire rapidly, so the families wouldn't be in the ICU for very long. This partially solved the problem of patients dying without their families being allowed to say goodbye properly, but it seemed coercive to me.

Prayer 143 (September 10, 2020)
Lord, I pray for my kids.
I tried to be a good Christian Dad to them, taught your word when they were little, but it seems to me the world is always challenging their faith.
Say the word and their faith will survive.
They are looking for peace – I pray they find it through you.
Good Shephard, you never lose any of your sheep.
Don't let my kids ever be lost away from you.
Help me and Jean show them the right way,
in accordance with your will. We trust in you Good Shepherd!

I love and worry about my kids – both young adults now. Things are a lot more complicated for them than they were when we grew up in the 60s and 70s – I won't pretend I understand just *how* complicated.

Jean was the best mom they could possibly have had, but I sometimes wondered how good a father I was. I wasn't always home as often as I should have been, physically or mentally – a hazard of my profession. I didn't have the warmest shoulder to cry on. Working in the ICU all those years, witnessing the effects of the most horrible and lethal diseases had a way of wearing down my sympathy for the lesser injuries and illnesses of their childhoods.

Ultimately, neither chose a career in medicine. I didn't fault them for that, but I couldn't help but wonder whether that was a verdict on what they thought of my career choice and how it affected our family. But however distracted I might have been by my vocation, I never stopped caring about them, thinking about them, even while at work in the Covid ICU. "Kids – I love you. I'm proud of you both. Know that your mom and I pray for you all the time, even now that you're grown up!"

Prayer 144 (September 11, 2020)
Lord, I bow down at your feet.
I have no pride in what I am, except that I was made by you.
I have no legitimacy to cry out your name, except the holy blood your Son shed on my behalf.
I have no faith in my ability to do better tomorrow except through your Holy Spirit. Have mercy on me.

You lift me up.
You wash me clean and arraign me in proper garments.
You embrace me in your mighty arms.
Although my feet stumble, you make the path beneath them straight. You lead me back to your garden.
You make opportunity for me to love and forgive my brothers and sisters, for my own sake.
You proclaim your glory through your grace in my life.
Thank you Lord for choosing me.

September 13, 2020. *Bristlecone pines in the Wheeler Peak Grove, Great Basin National Park – photographed on a hiking trip with my daughter. Bristlecone pines are the oldest living things on Earth – some as old as 4800 years. Their longevity is partially attributed to the harsh conditions they survive in.*

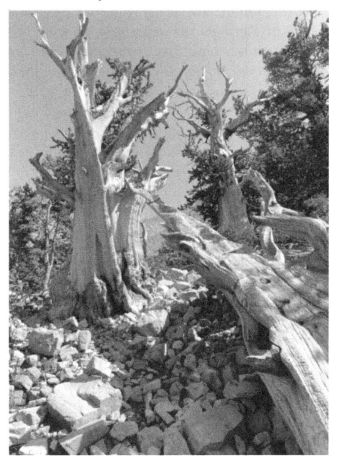

Prayer 145 (September 17, 2020)
Holy Savior Jesus, all-powerful creator, the searcher of my soul, the provider of my family, the hearer of my prayers – whose answer dictates my eternal future, who is completely pure, who is worthy

of all trust, who healed our impurity with his holy blood, who gifts us even our faith!
You made us to love us – make us worthy of your love by your grace.
We praise your holy name!

Prayer 146 (September 20, 2020)
I lay awake in the night, an emptiness chewing in the pit of my stomach, in the momentary realization that I am without direction as I simply survive each day, my future path dictated by my work schedule, surrounded by pitfalls on every side.
I'm like a lonely sheep wandering the wilderness.
Lord, flood this emptiness in my core.
Be my shepherd. Give my life purpose. Give my mind peace.
Love and faith arise from life's difficulties – therefore even these are a blessing.
Lead me down right paths, and call me righteous.
Protect me and my family from all evil and let me dwell in your shadow forever.

Prayer 147 (September 22, 2020)
Thank you Lord for every good thing you have provided for me today: waking up feeling good, thinking about my great kids, whispering goodbye to Jean as I head off to work, our nice home, driving to work safely in my comfortable car, my job helping patients and their families, my friends at work . . . my list goes on and on.
Don't know why you chose to save and bless me Lord, but I surely know that I am blessed and that all good things come from you.
Praise your holy name!

Rose was a previously healthy 51-year-old Navajo woman in our ICU with Covid pneumonia. There had been no significant change in her condition in the six days since she was intubated, and her care was becoming routine. Each day, I prayed for her, placing my gloved hand on her brow, maybe combing her hair back with my hand. I continued standard therapies, adjusted the ventilator and wrote my notes. But today, I stepped back and realized that Rose's chance of survival was fast diminishing along this course. "No change" was a bad thing in the ICU – *you had to get better to survive,* and Rose wasn't getting better.

She was on maximal ventilator settings. Her O2 sat actually *fell* when we proned her. She might still be a candidate for ECMO (extra-corporeal membrane oxygenation) – the advanced form of life support that we provided Anderson several months earlier. But if we were going to try it, we had to do so during the first week of mechanical ventilation – after that, the damage inflicted on her lungs by the high-pressure ventilator settings would have been too great. I needed to get consent from her family before starting the process of transferring Rose to an ECMO center, so I sat down at the nursing station and called Rose's mother, Lorena, from a landline.

"Hello?"

"Hi – is this Lorena?"

"Yes?"

"This is Dr. Eckshar from the hospital; I'm taking care of your daughter Rose."

"Uh, OK."

"Lorena, I wanted to give you a report on how Rose is doing and also ask you an important question about a treatment I think might help her."

"OK?"

"I'm sorry to tell you this, but Rose's situation is looking very serious. She is fighting for her life despite the ventilator and all the medicine we are giving her. I think she needs to go on a stronger sort of life support – a heart-lung machine called ECMO."

"Is that the same as a ventilator?"

"No. Rose has already *been* on a ventilator all this past week. It's not strong enough life support for her anymore." (*Insert my clumsy attempt to describe ECMO and how it's different than just a ventilator to Lorena*)

"So then, ECMO *is* a ventilator?" (*at this point, I have to admit, I had a brief unkind thought about Lorena*)

"No, Lorena, it's different and *stronger* than a ventilator."

Lorena paused as though trying to absorb it all, then surprisingly changed the subject – at first, I thought her mind was wandering, simply losing track of the ECMO conversation, which didn't seem to be getting anywhere.

"Rose is the *last* of my girls – my youngest. I already lost my other three daughters." (*Although, as it turns out, not due to Covid*).

"You lost your other three daughters?! Oh, I'm so sorry, Lorena."

She coughed weakly.

"Are you OK?"

"Yeah. My husband and I had Covid too – we just got out of the hospital last week."

"Are you better now?"

"We are OK . . . Rose has a son – 15 years old."

"Oh Lorena, I'm so sorry. I see even more now how important it is that we do the best job we possibly can for Rose."

"We're praying for her, doctor. Go ahead. Do the ECMO."

"Thanks, Lorena . . . say, do you think we should pray together? – right now?"

"Yes."

"OK, maybe I can start." I started praying, feeling my way along, searching for the right words, but Lorena started praying out loud, too, at the same time as me, drowning me out.

"Oh Jesus! Ohh Lord! Ohhh JESUS!"

My soft-spoken prayer was a clumsily attempted kindness by a stranger – Lorena's prayer was an outpouring of spontaneous, genuine emotion, the yearning love of a mother for her last surviving daughter. After a while, she quit using words altogether and continued simply wailing. I shut up – there was nothing my words could add to Lorena's expression of heartfelt grief. It degenerated into helpless sobbing as I silently held the phone in my shaking hand. Truth be told, I started crying too. [*Don't get the wrong impression that I'm one of these guys that's always crying. Before the pandemic, I don't think I had wept since high school.*]

I felt a physical presence close behind me and I was embraced in a bearhug around my shoulders from behind. I had no idea who it was, and didn't care – *I needed that hug.* I didn't look around to see who until a few minutes later when Lorena's prayer ended and we hung up the phone. My shoulder-hugger was one of our new ICU nurses, Zack. He had only worked with us in the ICU for about a month.

"Zack – thanks for that hug, brother – whew, I needed it!" I smiled.

"It's OK, doc. I wasn't going to let you have to pray for that lady alone."

Prayer 148 (September 23, 2020)
You say you see no hope.
You say you see no reason we should dream
that the world would ever change.
You say the love is foolish to believe;
'cause they'll always be some crazy
with an army or a knife,
to wake you from your daydream –
put the fear back in your life.

Look, If someone wrote a play
to just to glorify what's stronger than hate,
would they not arrange the stage
to look as if the hero came too late?
He's almost in defeat.
It's looking like the evil side will win.
So on the edge of every seat,
from the moment that the whole thing begins.

But it's Love who mixed the mortar,

and it's Love who stacked these stones
and it's Love who made the stage here,
although it looks like we're alone.
In this scene, set in shadows,
like the night is here to stay –
there is evil cast around us,
but it's Love that wrote the play
For in this darkness, Love can show the way.
[Lyrics to "Show the Way" by one of my favorite psalmists, David Wilcox. *I capitalized the word "Love" in this song, which I interpret as the name for God in this song.*]

The summer surge was fast waning from a peak of over 900 cases a day; now below 200. On September 23, 2020, our ICU was empty of Covid patients. All had either transferred out (like Rose) or died.

I thought about what it would be like to start your nursing career like Zack had – during the worst ICU catastrophe in history (given that we didn't have ICUs back during the Spanish influenza pandemic). Many new nursing grads must surely have doubted their vocation during Covid. I tried to encourage all the young nurses in our ICU that things almost certainly would get better if they could just make it through. Then they would have war stories to tell the newbies who came along after Covid. With God's grace, they might never face something so professionally challenging for the whole rest of their lives.

Prayer 149 (September 26, 2020)
A lot of earthly devices plague us Lord – our own inventions.
But you gave us love, the gift that overcomes them all.
Thank you Lord for the love of my wife and kids, for the love of my Christian brothers and sisters, for the love of my friends from all walks of life, – some of whom live only now in memory – for the love of the nurses and cafeteria staff and respiratory therapists, for the love of patients and their families, for the love of people I hardly know who were kind to me at a store or restaurant or on a

telephone helpline – people who just smiled at me when we shared an elevator.

You gave us a mighty shield against evil Lord – help me not forget to use it every chance I get.

Vincenzo, *the 63-year-old man who received prolonged life support despite requesting DNR status, posted a picture of himself smiling, skinny, sun-tanned and sun-glassed at the Chapel of the Holy Cross in the red rocks of Sedona, Arizona*

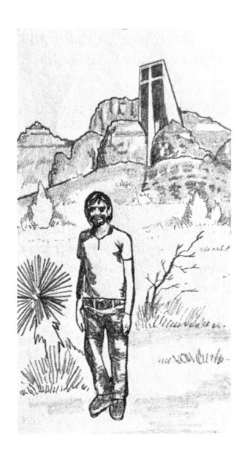

Vincenzo's daughter posted this message: "My father, was a former Covid patient for almost two months and we just wanted to let you know he is doing very well! He just recently celebrated his birthday and our family is so happy that he was given a second chance at life. Thank you to all your staff for saving his life! My whole family is filled with immense gratitude for all their sacrifices and for helping so many people during this terrible time. To our healthcare heroes on the front lines of Covid, working tirelessly to save lives, thank you for all you continue to do. Patients, families and our entire community are grateful for you!"

I realized Vincenzo would not have made it if it weren't for his family rescinding his DNR order. It was one of those decisions that you couldn't judge until its consequences became clear over time. *Thanks God for blessing that difficult decision.*

Prayer 150 (September 30, 2020, for our kids)
Lord, we thank you from the bottom of our hearts for our Heaven-sent children.
Don't let their faith be limited by our less-than-perfect parenting. Say the word that their faith will stand and grow.
Provide for them Lord. Guard them against temptation – all the worldly devices of evil they have to face – things that weren't even invented when we were kids – things meant to drag them down in worry and make them lose hope in their future.
Lord, give them the wisdom and faith to shut those voices out and find your peace.

Although our unit was briefly free of Covid, it was still an ICU. We were not free from catastrophe. Today we admitted Melissa, a 32-year-old woman with massive internal bleeding associated with childbirth. She required replacement of her entire blood volume three times over, during attempts to control the bleeding, and emergency surgery to ligate the bleeding uterine arteries and relieve the pressure caused by the massive hematoma in her pelvis. She initially stabilized but suddenly passed out two days later, and was found to have a huge PE (pulmonary embolism) – a blood clot that likely originated in her legs or pelvis that broke free and travelled through her veins to impact her lungs. She was started on a strong blood thinner even though she nearly passed away from bleeding just a few days ago; PE was the most immediate threat to her life.

This morning, two days later, Melissa suddenly became comatose. A CT of her brain showed a massive hemorrhagic stroke. There was so much blood inside her skull that it was crushing her brain and our neurosurgeons rushed her to the OR to remove the back of her skull and as much of the hematoma as possible, to relieve the pressure.

Prayer 151 (October 3, 2020)
Jesus, you gave us this hope: "You will grieve but your grief will turn to joy.
A woman giving birth to a child has pain because her time has come, but when her baby is born she forgets the anguish because of her joy that a child is born into the world.
So with you. Now is your time of grief, but I will see you again and you will rejoice, and no one will take away your joy.
Very truly I tell you, my Father will give you whatever you ask in my name.
Ask and you will receive, and your joy will be complete."
Thank you for this hope.
We ask the Father, in your holy name, to deliver us!
[From John 16:20-24]

This morning, Melissa's neurological examination revealed no sign of consciousness, only the most primitive brainstem reflexes. The neurologist presented a grim prognosis: even if Melissa miraculously survived, she would experience severe neurological disability. After careful consideration, Melissa's husband, Paul opted for comfort care. "Melissa would never want to live like that." I agreed with his decision – thought that God had made his will pretty clear – not one medical intervention since her admission had accomplished anything positive for Melissa*.

Samantha and I conspired to bring baby Veronica – Melissa and Paul's newborn daughter – up to the ICU for Melissa to hold, so that mother and newborn could be together at least once in this world. Although babies were not typically allowed in the ICU, no one stood in the way.

Paul arrived. The post-partum nurses brought Veronica up, swaddled but alert, and placed her in the crook of Melissa's left arm. Sam touched me on the shoulder and pointed at the monitor – Melissa's heart rate gradually fell from 113 to 79 – then stabilized there. Even in a coma, Melissa could still feel the presence of her daughter, and her distress was comforted. We joined hands around the bed and all prayed together.

[*I was wrong in this pessimism. Nothing happens without God's purpose being realized. Our medical interventions had two great benefits: baby Veronica was born healthy and had one chance to feel her mother's warm embrace.]

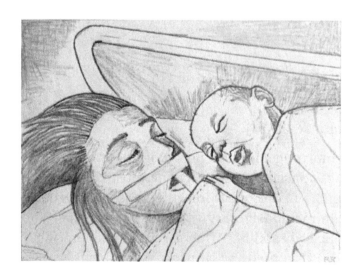

Prayer 152 (October 4, 2020)

Lord – give me a servant's heart.

Then the King will say to me: "Come, you who are blessed by my Father, inherit the kingdom prepared for you from the foundation of the world.

For I was hungry and you gave me food,

I was thirsty and you gave me drink,

I was a stranger and you welcomed me,

I was naked and you clothed me,

I was sick and you visited me,

I was in prison and you came to me."

Then I will answer him, saying, "Lord, when did I see you hungry and feed you, or thirsty and give you drink?

And when did I see you a stranger and welcome you, or naked and clothe you?

And when did I see you sick or in prison and visit you?"

And the King will answer: "Truly, I say to you, as you did it to one of the least of these my brothers, you did it to me."

[A personal application of Matthew 25:34-40]

Prayer 153 (October 5, 2020)

Praise the Lord my soul.

Blessed are those whose hope is in the Lord their God.

He is the maker of Heaven and Earth, the sea, and everything in them.

He upholds the cause of the oppressed.

He feeds the hungry and sets prisoners free.

He gives sight to the blind and lifts up those that are broken down.

The Lord loves the righteous, watches over the foreigner, and sustains the fatherless and the widow.

The Lord reigns forever, our God for all generations.

Praise the Lord my soul!

[Psalm 146 abbreviated]

Prayer 154 (October 6, 2020)

The Lord is good to all, and his mercy is over all that he has made.

The Lord is righteous in all his ways and kind in all his works.
The Lord is near to all who call on him in truth.
He fulfills the desire of those who fear him; he hears their cry and
saves them.
My mouth will shout the praise of the Lord, and let all I am bless his
holy name forever and ever.
[Another prayer based on Psalm 145]

I interacted with two very different families this day. The first comprised the wife and daughter of a 43-year-old man who went by "Willy" admitted with a hemorrhagic stroke. Willy weighed 439 pounds, had untreated high blood pressure, and drank a six-pack a day. When Willy arrived in the ED, his blood pressure was an astounding 254/136 – *high enough to impress even an old ICU veteran like me.* His mental status rapidly declined upon arrival due to the expanding hemorrhage in his brain demonstrated by CT. I emergently intubated him and the neurosurgeons performed an emergency craniotomy (opening of his skull for surgical evacuation of blood) to relieve perilously high intracranial pressure. Post-op, Willy went into severe delirium tremens due to alcohol withdrawal, making his hypertension spike erratically whenever we tried to lift sedation to perform neurological examinations.

Each time I sought communication with his family, their questions were accusatory: "Why didn't Willy get to surgery sooner?" (he was in the operating room within an hour of admission). "Why did they let Willy's blood pressure go up so high? (he was on six different antihypertensive medications, but his blood pressure was spiking because he was in alcohol withdrawal). "Why didn't you get Willy's MRI sooner?" (the scan was delayed because of his weight – the scanner table wasn't rated to carry over 400 lbs).

The follow-up MRI showed that Willy had suffered multiple new strokes in addition to the original hemorrhage seen on the CT scan. The neurosurgeons, neurologist and I all notified his family that, unfortunately, Willy had no chance of meaningful recovery. We suggested comfort care. The family flatly refused to discuss this further with us. They asked for a "second opinion" – *which actually would have constituted a* fourth *opinion, if you count me, the neurologist and the neurosurgeon –* from a neurologist not associated with our hospital. His wife was wearing a neckless with a cross hanging from it, but I didn't ask to pray with her. In retrospect, doing so might have healed our relationship, but praying together just didn't feel sincere at the time. So I failed Willy's family in that, and they never developed any trust in me or our team.

The second family was the husband and daughter of a 62-year-old woman named Rita, who had been intubated 14 days for Covid pneumonia – one of only a few we currently had left in the unit at the time. She had progressively deteriorated despite receiving all standard therapies. Without going into all her details – *which you can likely guess by this point* – take my word, it was looking hopeless. When I saw her that day, I felt with 100% certainty that she would not survive. I couldn't pray for God to heal her anymore without feeling I was rejecting his clearly-expressed decision:

Rita, I hope you don't mind me praying for you.
I pray for you in the holy name of God.
You are his daughter, and he loves you more than anyone here on Earth, and he is completely in charge of what happens to you.
I pray for you in complete trust that whatever he has in store for you will be better than anything here on Earth we can imagine.

I called Rita's husband, Phil and her daughter to talk about the situation. I had little previous direct contact with them, although they were aware of how poorly things were going through daily discussions with the nurses.

"Phil, I just want you to know that we tried hard for Rita – we gave her every treatment shown to help Covid patients, and even one...."

Phil: "Let me stop you right there Doc. We trust you. And we know how hard you tried – the nurses told us each day. Rita can't go on like this. It's time to let her be at peace. The nurses told us all about comfort care – I think that's what Rita would want."

"OK Phil. Sorry it's come to this." I paused momentarily, "Would Rita want us to pray with her?"

Phil smiled, "You know, doc, I don't think she would mind. She never was one much for prayer. But I think she would be OK with it if she knew *you* wanted to." So I did.

Prayer 155 (October 7, 2020)
Lord, thanks for giving us challenges that we cannot overcome on our own.
I have prayed for you to deliver me from some of these, but those that I have been forced to struggle through have shown me how much we all need to depend on you and each other.
Thanks for letting us know you are always around, and that anything difficult we encounter has only been allowed to challenge us in accordance with your will, for our benefit, so that we can learn to lean on the Holy Spirit and love each other.
Love and faith arise from lives difficulties – therefore even these are a blessing!

Prayer 156 (October 8, 2020)
Our Father –God of forgiveness, you sent your only Son to live and die among us, to set us free from the merciless snares of sin and death.
Forgive what we cannot forgive; heal what we dare not face; grant humility where we take refuge in false pride.
Grant us singleness of heart and a steadfast spirit, through Christ our Lord.

I had one of the most frustrating family meetings of my career today. I met with the wife and son of Dr. Langleiden, a 97-year-old retired surgeon, admitted after he choked on his breakfast, coded, and was intubated for aspiration pneumonia (having essentially inhaled eggs and sausage into his lungs). Dr. Langleiden had been bedbound for years, unable to speak or move his limbs as a consequence of multi-infarct dementia (a multitude of strokes resulting in dementia). He could chew and swallow if the food was placed in his mouth, but current events proved even that meager pleasure was no longer safe for him. He was cachectic as a concentration camp victim, his limbs wasted and contracted. When the nurses rolled him over to examine his backside, as per routine, they found a huge pressure ulcer had eroded through his paper-thin skin and few remaining muscle fibers, exposing his sacral bones to their horrified inspection. In my expressed opinion, no good outcome could possibly result from ongoing mechanical ventilation, which at this point was only prolonging the poor man's agony.

But when I met with Dr. Langleiden's wife and son, they were completely impassive in the face of his disastrous prognosis as I described it to them. At one point, his wife interrupted me to say that she liked the painting on the wall behind me. She wasn't paying any attention to what I was telling her about her husband, *and she wanted me to know it!* They were calmly adamant that Dr. Langleiden receive every available aggressive therapy and remain full code. I asked if he had a living will, and they reluctantly admitted he did but countered by asking why I would need to see it! "So that we could honor his wishes" was not a sufficient answer for them. They informed me they would produce the document *only* when they thought it was applicable. I couldn't change their minds, but I also knew in my heart that I would *not* be the one to break Dr. Langeleiden's ribs in the act of CPR. I couldn't imagine he could possibly want me to do that. I had to draw the line somewhere.

After some discussion about this case, our group proposed a hospital policy to deal with situations in which doctors and nurses are asked to provide care that they feel is immoral.

It was eventually implemented after many months of legal hand-wringing, employing a series of ethical safeguards but allowing caregivers some recourse to refuse to offer ACLS when it clearly violated the principle of non-maleficence (that doctors and nurses should never harm the patient). We used this policy only in extreme cases, about once a year.

When I was taught medical ethics back in the 80s, the cornerstones of decision-making included consideration of the patient's right to choose, benefits and harms to the patient, and social justice. The rights *of nurses and doctors* were never considered part of the equation. Partially because of this, one of the main contemporary causes of burnout is the moral distress healthcare workers suffer from being repeatedly forced to administer harmful therapies at the request of unreasonable surrogates.

Prayer 157 (October 11, 2020)
Have mercy on me God, according to your steadfast love, according to your abundant mercy, blot out my transgressions.
Wash me thoroughly from my iniquity and cleanse me from my sins.
For I know my transgressions and my sin is ever before me."
[David's cry, based on Psalm 51 – shared by Tom D.]

Prayer 158 (October 16, 2020)
Author of life, we praise you. Maker of purpose, we thank you.
Giver of peace, we implore you.
Don't let us waste our time on Earth Lord.
Show us the right path you prepared for us before we were born.
Don't let the world lead us astray.
Let us sleep in peace each night knowing we did the work you apportioned us.
This I ask of you – that you would put your mighty arm on my shoulders someday and say, "Job well done, good and faithful servant." [Matthew 25:23]

I accepted the transfer of a 20-year-old woman, Roxanna,

who presented to an outlying hospital coughing up blood. She tested negative for Covid, but a CT scan showed a large PE (pulmonary embolism). Although her vital signs were stable at the time, a blood clot this large in her lungs could become precipitously life-threatening unless properly treated.

Although it was 4 pm, Roxanna looked like she was asleep in her hospital bed when I walked in to examine her. The first thing she said when I woke her was that she needed something strong for pain – her chest hurt when coughed. She was irritable and fixated on getting pain relief, and I could tell I wasn't going to be able to get much more than the most rudimentary history from her until I took care of that. I asked a few basic questions, which she curtly answered, looked her over, then went out to check for any past medical records in the EMR (none) and to call her mom Linda, for which Roxanna had granted permission.

Linda told me that Roxanna had been smoking methamphetamine and fentanyl regularly for about a year and that she was a mother of a newborn baby boy and a 4-year-old girl, both in the custody of Child Protective Services. *The recent birth of her son was likely the cause of her blood clot; peripartum blood clots usually originated in the deep veins of the left leg, which are sometimes compressed by the gravid uterus.*

As I briefly ruminated on the pathophysiology of the blood clot, Linda started crying, bringing me back to the present. Roxanna had stubbornly argued with her mom about coming into the hospital – Linda had to *beg her* to come in. Roxanna was already texting her mom that she "needed a fix" and was threatening to check herself out of the hospital AMA (against medical advice).

"Doctor – please don't let her leave . . . you have to keep her!"

"I'll do what I can to get her to stay. But I can't legally *force her* to stay."

"*Please,* doctor – do whatever you can; Roxanna is my baby girl . . ." she broke down sobbing.

"I'll do my best for your daughter Linda. I promise."

After I got off the phone, I took Roxanna's nurse Lynn aside to come up with a game plan. Lynn looked doubtful: "Dr. Eckshar – She's already threatening to leave AMA!"

"Lynn, we both know she might be playing us about this pain issue, but if she leaves AMA, she's going to die. Are you OK if we give in to her regarding pain meds?" Lynn nodded. *I had trusted she would – she had strong empathy – her own daughter in college.* "Thanks. I'm going to write for fentanyl* 100 micrograms every three hours as needed for pain. We can go up a little if that doesn't work. Let's go along with her on any issues that we can, and try to get her to stay. And please get that heparin (blood thinner) started STAT, OK?"

I went back into the room to speak to Roxanna. "Roxanna, I wrote for some IV fentanyl for your chest pain – *no need to explain what fentanyl was.* Lynn is getting some for you now. Your CT scan shows a big blood clot in your lungs. It's dangerous and that's what's causing your chest pain. We are going to start you on some blood thinners to treat that. But you're going to need to stay here for –

"I need to go now," she interrupted with a stubborn look.

"Roxanna, you need to stay until we have this blood clot under control. Do you understand <u>you could die</u> if you leave here without treatment? Work with us, OK? We're on your side. Tell us what you need within reason, and we'll help make your stay tolerable. Your mom and your kids are counting on you."

Roxanna regarded me sullenly and nodded her head yes, with the subtlest of nods. I prayed to myself that she would let us do our job. Can't say why I didn't offer to pray with her – it just didn't feel right. I overthink that at times and I never got another chance.

[*Fentanyl is a strong narcotic pain killer akin to morphine; originally used in the operating room and ICU, it was now being illicitly mass-produced for purposes of abuse. Illicit fentanyl "M30" pills are widely available for sale for about 50 cents each.

With unstandardized doses and purity, a single pill could deliver a fatal overdose to an intolerant person, and regular fentanyl users also frequently die from the doses they believe they can tolerate. Fentanyl overdose is currently the number one cause of death in people 18-45 years of age, killing more young people than cancer, heart disease, and accidents.]

Prayer 159 (October 17, 2020)
Holy Spirit – help me in my weakness.
I don't even know what I ought to pray for; but intercede for me with thoughts that can't be expressed in human words.
The searcher of my heart knows your mind because you intercede for me in accordance with his will.
I know that in all things, God works for my good, since I seek him, I love him and I have been called – all according to his purpose.
[From Romans 8:26-27]

I was off from work but had awoken early thinking about Roxanna. I waited until 7 am – *there wouldn't be any new chart entries before then* – and accessed Roxanna's electronic chart remotely from home to see how she was doing. Viewing the chart this way was not the same as boots on the ground; I couldn't tell much. There were no new doctor's notes and no new lab results yet, but it was still early.

Around lunchtime, I checked again – still no new doctor's notes. *Strange.* I checked for morning labs – none. Did I forget to order morning labs for her? A frightening suspicion dawned on me. I opened the last note recorded in her chart from the previous night. It was brief, merely stating that Roxanna had checked herself out of the hospital AMA.

Prayer 160 (October 21, 2020)
For God alone my soul waits in silence; from him comes my salvation.
He alone is my rock and my fortress – I shall not be shaken.
All authority belongs to God, and to you Lord belongs steadfast love!

For you will render to man according to his faith!
[Psalm 62 abbreviated]

Prayer 161 (October 23, 2020)
Lord, hear our cry.
Even when our mouths are silent, our souls cry out to you.
Our happiness, our very lives here on Earth are so tenuous, so uncertain.
We would be even more afraid than we already are if we truly realized what a highwire we are trying to balance on; doing everything we can to make things turn out right.
You put that drive in us when you made us.
But Lord, we know we can't hack it.
Help us do our best Lord, but we place our trust not in ourselves, but in you.
You are our rock and our fortress and no earthly challenge we face can overcome you.

In the ICU, we might be alternately forced to provide futile care to an incapacitated 97-year-old man without any hope for a happy future, then denied the opportunity to provide life-saving treatment to a young mother with her entire adult life ahead of her. We are coerced accomplices in the irrational personal decisions of patients and their surrogates, doomed to take part in their mistakes and observe the predictably horrible outcomes. We maintain their autonomy at our own peril: the accumulated moral distress of participating in disastrous events that we are often powerless to alter.

Prayer 162 (October 29, 2020)
Lord, I was lying awake in bed last night and prayed for you to speak to me.
Tell me what to do today.
But then I just prayed for you to open my ears.
Your word is <u>always</u> around us if we only stop and listen.

I immediately heard: "Love each other as I loved you."
I don't know what that's going to look like today, but keep my eyes

sharp Lord, and help me recognize my chances to do the work of your kingdom today.

Our ICU census was up to 23, five with Covid pneumonia. Things were slowly heating up again for another round. The Winter surge was on its way.

Prayer 163 (October 30, 2020)
The Heavens stretch to hold you and deep cries out to deep saying:
"Nothing is beyond you!"
Time cannot contain you.
You fill eternity.
Sin can never stain you.
Death has lost its sting.
I cannot explain the way you came to love me, except to say that nothing is beyond you!
[Lyrics by Rich Mullins]

That night I dreamed I walked into a patient's room and found her prepped and awaiting surgery. We were in an operating room. I had never met the patient before, but it seemed entirely natural to push my way through the OR nurses surrounding the operating table and closely examine her internal organs. The skin and soft tissue of her chest wall and abdomen had already been incised down the midline and widely retracted so that all her internal organs were exposed. Her lungs were surrounded by spongy blobs of dead tissue, which I meticulously removed with forceps until the lungs were pink and healthy-looking. I watched them slowly and fully inflate with inspiration – *they looked fine now*. I looked down at the patient's spleen and liver when suddenly, the nurses began shouting to me that the patient was waking up.

I shouted, "Quick – give her 300 micrograms of fentanyl!"

"We don't have any fentanyl."

"Then 10 milligrams of Versed."

"We don't have any Versed."

"What *DO* you have?!"

"Nothing – we have nothing, doctor – we have no sedation drugs!" The patient was now fully awake, looking at me calmly over her exposed organs, taking things in impassively as I panicked.

"How the hell can you have set this patient up for surgery without any anesthesia drugs?!" The patient was listening avidly, clearly aware that something was going very wrong. I was frightening her – *I had to drop my voice, get myself under control.*

A nurse told me not to worry; it was all going to be OK now. The nurses would close. She took me by the elbow and led me away from the patient, out of the OR, confused as I could be.

I awoke sweaty, my pulse racing. My back ached. It took me a moment to realize I was at home in bed. I stretched and pulled my sheets off, didn't even try to figure out what the dream meant, except that I probably wouldn't be getting back asleep tonight. After a few minutes, I picked up my Kindle off the bedside table: 3:37 am. I had only a little more than an hour before I had to get up for work. I opened *True Grit* by Charles Portis and started reading.

WINTER SURGE 2020: HOPE

Prayer 164 (November 2, 2020)
Father, have mercy on America.
Forgive our many sins and soften the consequences
of our mistakes.
We have fallen away from you in many ways, but we are still a
land of Christians!
Help us stand up to that honor and become what a nation of
Christians should be.
Let our country give you honor and praise and treat each other as
brothers and sisters. Don't forsake us to the evil that divides us, but
hear our cry and lift us up.
Still one nation under God!

Prayer 165 (November 5, 2020)
On that day when evening had come Jesus said to them: "Let us go
across to the other side."
And leaving the crowd they took him with them in the boat.
And a great windstorm arose and the waves were breaking into the
boat so that the boat began to swamp.
But Jesus was in the stern asleep on the cushion.
And they woke him and said to him "Teacher do you not care that
we are perishing?" And he awoke and rebuked the wind and said to
the sea: "Peace! Be still!"
And the wind ceased and there was a great calm.
And he said to them "Why are you so afraid?
Have you still no faith?" [Mark 4:35-40]

My route to the hospital had been carefully optimized to
reduce driving stress – on a lucky day, I might make the entire
25-minute drive without encountering a single red light. I took
maximal advantage of the freeway HOV lane, unrestricted for
my use before 6 am. I would easily be off the freeway by then at

my current cruise control speed of 79 mph –by my reckoning, the speed that best balanced efficient use of my travel time and the risk of getting a speeding ticket. Chris Botti's smooth jazz trumpet provided a calming, mind-focusing soundtrack for the drive.

I pulled into the closest covered space outside the hospital and headed to the grill for breakfast, arriving just as they opened. I yelled hey to Yuri, and he nodded back, "Be with you in a minute, doc!" The guy in front of me was ordering an omelet.

"Could I please have a two-egg omelet with cheese, spinach, onions, and peppers?"

Yuri looked at him impassively, "You want mushrooms?"

The guy was apparently unprepared for that particular question; he looked confused, perhaps even afraid. "Umm . . ." *Like a deer in headlights.*

Yuri raised his eyebrows, "It is a simple question: Do you want mushrooms with your omelet?" – carefully enunciating each syllable.

The guy decided the best way to survive the interaction was to concede. "Yes. Sure. Put mushrooms in there too."

Yuri smiled ear to ear, "Now you're talking!"

I had to hide my grin, not wanting to embarrass the guy, but wondering if he even liked mushrooms. You didn't want to show any kind of indecision around Yuri. He didn't have time for it.

We had received a 52-year-old man named Stanton in transfer from the floor overnight. Admitted three days earlier with a kidney infection, he subsequently went into a severe form of alcohol withdrawal called "DTs" (delirium tremens) despite the provision of beer for him to drink with his hospital meals and at bedtime.

His DTs had exceeded the considerable tolerance of the floor nurses, requiring ICU transfer. This had more to do with the incredible personal bedside care an ICU nurse provides than any technology we offer.

Delirium tremens is a state of severe agitation, delusion, and hallucination that is oftentimes unpreventable, hugely complicating what might otherwise have been a simple hospitalization. Due to the attendant behavioral issues, it was especially hard on nurses. Isaiah drew the short straw, but he accepted the assignment as always without complaint. I was going through Stanton's EMR at a computer station just outside his room and overheard their interaction.

Stanton: "I gotta get up and go to the store. Go to the store!" – trying to get out of bed. "You sonuvabitch! You can't hold me here! I got rights! I'm a citizen of the United States of America! The greatest nation on Earth! You didn't even read me my rights!"

Isaiah calmly: "It's OK, Stanton. Lie back and relax. You're sick in the hospital, but you're going to be OK."

Stanton laughed: "I'm not in the hospital – I'm being illegally incarcerated in here! I wanna a lawyer! I got rights! I gotta go to the store!" Despite the soft restraints tethering Stanton's wrists to the sides of his bed (to prevent him from pulling his IVs out), he had contorted himself, squirming both legs off the right side of this bed. Isaiah gently lifted his legs and straightened them out in bed.

Stanton became momentarily calm: He looked Isaiah right in the eyes, his sensorium momentarily seemed to clear and he said "Hey Lonnie, Do you have any lip balm? My lips hurt."

Isaiah: "I'll get you some ice chips to suck on Stanton – that will help."

Isaiah fluffed Stanton's pillow and pulled the sheet up over him. As I entered the room for my examination, Isaiah took the opportunity to step out and get some charting done. Stanton kicked the sheet off, had a diarrheal bowel movement and started scissoring his legs back and forth, spreading it like peanut butter all over the insides of his thighs and the bedsheets.

There was nothing to do but continue my examination. But

I had to tell Isaiah about this "code brown" right afterward. Back when visitation was allowed, a family chancing into the room at such a moment would invariably complain about the poor care being delivered. The fact is, the nurses can't be at the bedside every minute that it takes to keep up with a patient in DTs. A few minutes later, Isaiah took the news with his typical good-humored exasperation. He gathered a washbasin, a deep stack of wash clothes and towels, and a paper filter full of coffee grounds* onto the bedside table, put on a pair of gloves, pulled the drapes and got to work. [*An old nursing trick to help control bad smells].

Prayer 166 (November 10, 2020)

Lord – Sometimes it seems only under great adversity will I turn to you.
I wonder if it is even possible to rekindle my reliance on you in the absence of catastrophe.

Yes; it is possible.
I can't, but you can.
My soul cries out to you.
Don't let me mess things up for myself again.
But keep me under your wings. Hide me in your temple.
Let me dwell in your house forever!

Isaiah had arranged a FaceTime call with Stanton's wife, Clarissa, so I could update her. She and their 14-year-old daughter appeared together. I was a little surprised, although I didn't know what I expected. They both came across smart and good-hearted, reminding me a little of our favorite neighbors. Stanton was a software engineer, and a decent father and husband, except for his drinking. He was making arrangements to enter an alcohol rehabilitation program when the urinary infection intervened. The discrepancy between Stanton's condition in the hospital and how his wife and daughter described him at home was remarkable. That he had such an apparently fine and loyal family struck me as something that would help me take better care of him.

Later in the day and unbeknownst to me, a 53-year-old man named Donovan presented to our ER complaining of persistent back pain from a minor motorcycle accident he was involved in five days previously. Incidentally, he was coughing a bit, and his O2 sat was 91%. A rapid Covid test and chest X-ray were both positive and Donovan was admitted to the general hospital ward for mild Covid pneumonia.

Prayer 167 (November 13, 2020)
Hear my cry Lord – have mercy upon me and answer me.
You have said, "Seek my face."
My heart answers, "Your face do I seek, hide not your face from me!"
Don't turn away from your servant Lord, you have been my help.
Do not forsake me, you who are my salvation!
For even if my family and friends forsake me, the Lord will take me in.

The Lord is my light and my salvation; whom shall I fear?
The Lord is the stronghold of my life; of whom shall I be afraid?
Though an army encamps against me, my heart shall not fear.
One thing I have asked of the Lord, that I will seek with all my heart: that I may dwell in the house of the Lord all the days of my life, to gaze upon the beauty of the Lord and inquire in his temple.
For he will hide me in his shelter.
In days of trouble he will lift me high upon a rock and my head will be lifted up.
I believe that I shall look upon the goodness of the Lord in the land of the living!
[Another prayer based on Psalm 27]

Today I saw a patient named Preston, an 81-year-old man with primary bacterial pneumonia (*not* Covid pneumonia) who was doing well on his second day of mechanical ventilation. That morning, he got ahold of his ETT and pulled it out despite soft wrist restraints*. As is often the case, the patient was correct in his decision to self-extubate. He was breathing room air without any supplemental oxygen when I saw him just afterward. He was an alert, onery, leather-skinned old guy who looked like (and was) a long-time smoker. He could have been one of the Marlboro men back in the day. A few hours later, I checked back in on him and wrote transfer orders out to the floor – *he didn't look like he needed ICU care anymore.* About fifteen minutes after writing the orders, I had a feeling that I should amend them and order electronic heart monitoring on him to continue after he left the ICU, although there was no objective reason to do so. His heart seemed fine. [*Patients are restrained when the nurses determine that they pose a significant risk to their own safety by unintentionally pulling out essential items such as their IV lines or ETT. Highly motivated patients sometimes get around this by contorting their body position. If they can't bring their hand up to the ETT, they can sometimes bring the ETT to their hand by bending their neck and torso towards the bedrail.*]

Prayer 168 (November 14, 2020)
On the day of my trouble, I seek the Lord.
My hands are stretched out to you; my soul refuses to be comforted.
But then I said, "Let me remember the years of blessing from the Lord . . . his mighty deeds and the wonders he has worked."
Has his steadfast love ever ceased?
Has his mercy been forgotten?
Your way, O Lord, is holy! You are the God of miracles.
Your mighty arm reaches out and saves your children.
We know you will not forget us today and nothing can stand in the way of your loving plan.
Your word is law. All praise to you!
[Adaptation of Psalm 77]

The day after Preston had transferred out, the code bells went off in the telemetry monitoring unit. I was on call, so I grabbed my P100 and ran up there.

When I arrived, I took my typical position at the head of

the bed, from where I could manage the airway, see the heart monitor and give orders to the other code team members. Looking at the patient from that strange visual perspective, above and behind him, and being preoccupied with running the code, it took me a few minutes before I recognized Preston. But there he was – coding!

I re-intubated Preston and followed ACLS protocol for twenty minutes without regaining so much as a single heartbeat. It was highly unlikely at this point that he could be resuscitated by any further intervention. I asked if any of the fifteen or so people in the room had any further suggestions before I "called the code" (called it quits). The room went silent – no suggestions – we had tried everything. "OK – stop CPR" The person giving chest compressions stopped, stood back and took a deep breath. The monitor was flatline.

"If you guys don't mind, let's observe a moment of silence for Preston," I said, laying my hand on his arm. The room got very quiet for a moment. Then I looked up at the monitor, which had begun chirping.

Preston's heart had resumed beating on its own. "Check for a pulse, Check for a pulse!" *Checking . . . checking . . .* there it is! Faint but now a bit stronger. "Check a blood pressure; grab some Levophed!" Preston had spontaneously returned to life!

Preston's floor nurse later told me he seemed fine all morning, just had a little nausea after breakfast and hadn't reported any shortness of breath or chest pain. "We thought he was going to go home later today. The monitoring station notified us he was bradying-down (a plummeting heart rate that sometimes heralds code arrest) and when I ran in to check on him, he was out."

I met Preston's wife outside the room and told her about the code and Preston's current condition. She was badly shook-up; they had been married 44 years. Over the next week, Preston regained consciousness and was eventually transferred to a skilled nursing facility. His code arrest was presumptively attributed to having unwitnessed aspiration of vomit into his windpipe. Another lesson in humility: I called Preston dead, but God said not yet!

Prayer 169 (November 18, 2020)
As far as my understanding goes, no human understands why our consciousness moves inexorably forward through time*.
But your greatest gifts, all-powerful Father, help us understand your will, and to know your will is to possess wisdom.
You have given us forgiveness, through your greatest sacrifice, so that we can be free of guilt for our past.
You have given us faith so that we don't have to worry about our future; so we can live in the present moment, as you made us to do.
Help me fully accept faith and forgiveness, and live in the moment today, with your love in my heart.

[*Steven Hawking addresses this in his book "A Brief History of Time." Although he presented explanations that his fellow geniuses probably understood, none of them made sense to me. I think one thing that makes it hard for us to understand God is that he is conscious at all points of time simultaneously – past, present and future. So he doesn't have to interfere with free will by "predicting" what we are going to do. He is conscious of the future now and can see what we are going to do.*]

Prayer 170 (November 20, 2020)
I was looking at one of David's last acts as king in 2 Samuel 23. The Lord was angry with Israel and gave David a choice between several punishments. David chose pestilence (disease) because the outcome was in God's hands rather than in the hands of his human enemies – essentially betting on God's mercy. Seventy thousand Israelites died in just a few days, but God held back further calamity and accepted David's sacrifice in propitiation for the sins of Israel.

Lord, we have caused a deadly problem for ourselves, but even though our actions deserve your wrath, we trust in your mercy Father God, as David did.
And we have a much much more pleasing sacrifice than the one

David offered – the sacrifice of your beloved Son!
How much more will our faith in Christ's blood make our relationship with you right! And you will lift us up again.
We praise you Father God!
We are so blessed that our fate is in your hands and none other!

Our ICU census had reached 26 (100% of the maximum safe census) again, 12 with Covid pneumonia. We would have been flabbergasted to know that the winter surge would henceforth continuously exceed what we originally thought was our maximum safe census for almost 100 consecutive days through the end of February.

Carlos called to tell me his brother Mike was hospitalized for Covid pneumonia. Mike resided in a small skilled nursing facility (SNF) in Chicago. Thirty-four of 37 of his fellow residents had Covid. Mike eventually recovered, but 14 of his fellow residents died in the outbreak. Fourteen of 37 – *that's 38% mortality!* Another example how lethal Covid could be in vulnerable populations. An uncertain number of healthcare workers who worked in Mike's SNF were also infected. Two nurses ended up on ventilators and only one survived.

Prayer 171 (November 24, 2020)
In God I trust and I am not afraid.
What can the world do to me?
I lift up thanks to you, for you have delivered me from death and my feet from stumbling, so that I may walk before God in the light of life.

Now my heart, O God, is steadfast.
Awaken, my soul! I will praise you, Lord, among all people for your love is great, reaching to the Heavens.
Your faithfulness reaches the skies.
Be exalted O God, above the Heavens and let your glory reign over all the Earth! [Psalms 55-57 abbreviated]

I texted the prayer above to Carlos. He was on call

that night for a 60-bed hospital in the western suburbs of Chicago, overrun with Covid patients. He was later paged at 3:45 am to assume care of a 56-year-old Polish man named Stanley, who had Covid pneumonia, had coded five times and now was comatose and in refractory shock. Stanley had been managed by an ultramodern healthcare team: a remote telehealth intensivist and an on-site ICU nurse practitioner, who had managed to keep him barely alive while avoiding coming to terms with his impending death. They consulted Carlos because it looked like a temporary stalemate had been achieved between his death process and life support. Time to hand things over to an old-fashioned ICU doc. Carlos was taking responsibility for withdrawing the futile care and treating Stanley's family humanely, tasks which he was better suited to accomplish.

Carlos called Stanley's Polish-speaking-only wife Sophie and daughter Mirielle through an interpreter. He introduced himself. Sophie cried softly as Carlos described the untenable situation. Mirielle spoke of Stanley's life and his love of family. Carlos told Sophie and Mirielle that they couldn't code Stanley anymore. Mirielle asked if they could come to be with him, but Carlos explained the no-visitation policy. When she asked if there wasn't *anything* else they could do, it dawned on Carlos that they could pray. Carlos pulled up the prayer text on his cellphone and started reciting it in English, asking the interpreter to translate. She interrupted, "I already have this prayer on my phone – it is from Psalm 55."

Carlos described what happened next: "She read Psalm 55 in a lovely Polish voice. It sounded like a Christmas Carol. As the family softly cried, their hearts breaking, snow was falling outside, illuminated by moonlight. The prayer offered spiritual hope when there was no earthly hope. Stanley's soul was in the Lord's hands. All four of us felt it. Sophie and Mirielle thanked the interpreter and me. Afterwards, as I rolled over in bed to try to get another hour of sleep before the start of my workday, I thought: *this is what Christ tried to teach us –*

that we are here to love one another.

Prayer 172 (November 26, 2020)
Lord, thanks for all my tomorrows.
No matter how badly I mess up, you let me put it all behind me.
Can't change the past, but I know you forgive a contrite heart and
I can always start all over and try to do better tomorrow.
But that wouldn't work either, except for your Holy Spirit to guide
me!
What a hopeless mess of sin and guilt and regret I would be
without you.
But I can take a deep breath and let go of all that because of your
sacrifice on my behalf. Praise your holy name!

Our ICU census reached 37 patients (140% of our previous maximum safe census), 26 with Covid pneumonia.

Donovan's pneumonia progressed quickly over 48 hours and was now requiring a BiPAP mask with 90% oxygen. He was transferred up to the unit and by the next day required intubation. But within 24 hours, he seemed to rebound, self-extubated and was looking pretty strong. He was back on BiPAP but alert and able to eat some during brief interludes on a high-flow nasal cannula (you can't get food to your mouth while wearing a BiPAP mask). Donovan had big muscles and was tatted up; it made me think he might tough Covid out.

I was working long call, which meant that I picked up cross-coverage on my partners' patients in the afternoon. One of these patients, Mia, was a 36-year-old wife and mother of five young children. She didn't have any particular risk factors for severe Covid, but her course was treatment-resistant and relentlessly downhill. After 21 days on the ventilator, she reached the highest levels of life support our hospital could provide. The ECMO centers in our area were completely overwhelmed and not accepting transfers, *not even a 36-year-old mom!* We expected Mia could die on any given day now; we were each just hoping it wouldn't happen on our shift.

Mia's husband, Brent understood the situation and begged to come visit her, but as mentioned earlier, our strict visitation policy stipulated that the the family could only visit if they decided to withdraw life support. We were recommending comfort care for Mia anyway, but this visitation policy was embarrassing to explain. It seemed coercive to me – almost like we were twisting Brent's arm into accepting comfort care.

Brent half-heartedly agreed to our terms, drove in and asked for a little time to sit by Mia before "letting her go". After 90 minutes of holding Mia's hand and crying silently at her bedside, Brent came out and announced he couldn't do it – couldn't give up on her. He still wanted everything done. It crossed my mind that he might have just pulled a fast one, but I silently applauded him for having gotten around our inhumane policy. A husband or wife ought to have a right to be together before the end without calling it quits.

Although Brent was still requesting full-court press, Mia had deteriorated badly and it would require a miracle for her to survive the day no matter what we did. Her O2 sats fell into the 70s, then by the end of my shift, into the 60s. There didn't seem to be anything left we could do about it. I made sure her sedation and pain medication were adequate. She couldn't possibly last much longer, and it almost seemed cruel to prolong her struggle, but the thought crossed my mind to recheck her chest X-ray. I ordered one with some misgivings.

The chest X-ray, done just about the time Joyce arrived for her night shift, showed *both* of Mia's lungs had ruptured and collapsed – *something I had seen only once before in my career.* I explained the situation to Joyce. Neither of us was sure what to do; it seemed Mia would certainly die whether we placed chest tubes or not. But Brent had specifically asked us to do *everything* for Mia and we decided to stick with that plan, as futile as it seemed. Mia was only 36 and she had children. She passed away during the placement of the second chest tube. We told Brent the truth that we never gave up and kept fighting for Mia right to the very end.

The Covid unit had now grown to fill our entire ICU: our very last ICU beds having been converted to Covid beds, with IV pumps and ventilator control panels wired up outside the rooms.

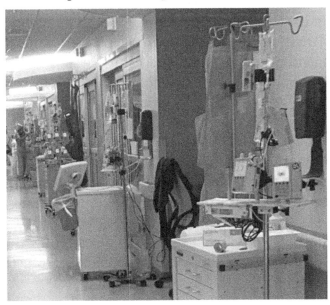

Prayer 173 (November 28, 2020)

Lord Jesus, loving Father, Creator of the Universe, Almighty Ruler of all time and space, who conquered death, we lift up your name in joy, in complete confidence that no puny source of evil, no unkind word, no setback, no shortage, no illness, no accident, no financial loss, no dictator, no war, nor any act of man or nature can ever separate us from your love, or change the happy future you have prepared for us.

Give us the faith today Lord to fully accept this fundamental truth.

Thanksgiving was turning into a nightmare. The service was over 40 patients (and would stay that way for the next 3 months). To put this in perspective, we had only reached a census as high as 26 patients once in all of 2019. All but a handful of our patients had severe Covid pneumonia. The ICU had become an overflowing Covid disaster response unit; boxes of various Covid PPE, ventilator control panels, and top-heavy IV poles outside every room – the patients virtually indistinguishable in their proning beds; or when those ran out, lying on their bellies face-down in bed on ventilators.

Each interminable long call shift was a unremitting adrenaline-pounding series of emergencies. On November 28, I saw 25 patients with life-threatening Covid pneumonia. I ran two codes and performed emergency chest tube surgery on two Covid patients with collapsed lungs. There was zero time for anything but rushing from one catastrophe to the next. Between emergencies, I went from room to room, quickly assessing each patient to determine whether they were likely to be next. It was like residing in an M.C. Escher woodcut – a never-ending Mobius passage with endless rooms filled with dying Covid patients, their identities blurring together into singularity.

My phone pinged – a text from one of my Bible study brothers: *Beloved, do not be surprised at the fiery trial when it comes upon you to test you, as though something strange was happening to you. But rejoice insofar as you share Christ's sufferings, that you may also rejoice and be glad when his glory is revealed* [1 Peter 4:12–13]." Good timing!

I entered the room of a new admit, Isabella, an 89-year-old African American woman with Covid pneumonia, afraid of what I would find. She was receiving oxygen by a high-flow nasal cannula, silent and thin as a skeleton. When I introduced myself to her apparently unconscious form, she surprised me by speaking.

"Cold."

Taken aback, I pulled her blankets up, which had bunched up about her knees.

"No," she croaked – "Something cold – *to drink!*"

I couldn't give her water. We had to keep her stomach empty in case we had to intubate her. "I'll bring you some ice chips." I brought back a cup of ice and a plastic spoon and Isabelle greedily accepted the ice chips I fed her*. Her voice cleared a little and she became more animated.

"What I really want is something ice-cold to *drink*."

"Well, we can't give you drink anything just yet, Isabella – are the ice chips OK for now?"

"I suppose," she cracked a subtle smile, "what I could *really* go for is an ice-cold Corona beer!" Twenty years melted away from her appearance.

That warmed my heart. I thought maybe I could relax just for a few minutes and enjoy joking around with her. "And what would you like to order to eat with that, ma'am?"

She perked up a little more: "I'll have a T-bone steak!"

"And how would you like that done, madame?"

"Well-done. I don't want to see any blood!" She scrunched up her face.

"OK, I understand; my wife likes her steak the same way. Baked potato?"

"Yes – with everything – sour cream *and* butter!"

"Salad?"

She made a face. "Nothing green!"

For a moment there, I felt human again, no longer a zombie. My ice-cold hands were warming up. Isabella was still a human being. This deathly-ill, elderly lady had turned the tables on her doctor – *she was so full of Holy Spirit, she was healing me!*

[*Bringing ice water to a thirsty patient and bringing warm blankets to a cold patient are two of my favorite things to do at work. I attend to these personally; ICU doctors have few such opportunities to bring instant alleviation of suffering!]*

Prayer 174 (December 2, 2020)
And I heard a loud voice from the throne saying, "Behold, the dwelling place of God is with man.
He will dwell with them, and they will be his people, and God

himself will be with them as their God."
[Revelation 21:3]
Thank you merciful and loving Father – having created the majestic breath of the universe, yet you have chosen to be with us and care for us on our tiny world in our time of trouble.
We praise you. Protect us today Lord.
Keep our families safe from evil. We put our trust in you!

Our census kept rising – no idea how high it might go. Because of the large number of licensed ICU beds at our hospital, the only thing limiting admissions from the statewide Covid triage system was the availability of nurses. The capacity of physicians was not considered at all – it was apparently assumed to be limitless. In order to take care of as many patients as possible, our hospital had made financial incentives to attract nursing "travelers" from across the country to come to work with us temporarily. This provided many unfamiliar faces in the unit. Unfortunately, every other hospital in the United States was doing the same thing, so the result was that the influx of traveling nurses was offset by the efflux of our nurses traveling elsewhere.

Almost all our nurses that traveled eventually ended up back in our ICU, expressing appreciation for "how good we had it here." But besides our camaraderie, coming back here wasn't an easy sell. Our nurses were stretched to 3:1 patient care assignments; that is, each nurse had to juggle three deathly ill Covid patients at once. Under normal circumstances, almost every one of these patients would have received 1:1 nursing care since a nurse could be expected to spend the entirety of their 12-hour shift continuously attending to a single patient's ICU needs. Now they had to play bop-a-mole with three patients at a time – a highly stressful and exhausting job.

Donovan had slowly faded and lapsed into agitated confusion. Now subdued and lethargic, he didn't look so tough anymore. He required reintubation, his kidneys began to shut down and he developed secondary bacterial pneumonia. Unknown to me at the time, Donovan's younger sister Nora had now also been admitted with Covid pneumonia. I would meet her only briefly about a week later.

I looked forward to seeing Isabella. But when I examined her, she was despondent and I couldn't cheer her up again. "I'm old, tired of all this," she waved her thin arms around, fluttering the IV lines, telemetry monitoring cables and oxygen tubing. That was the last time I ever talked to her. Over the next few days, Isabella became progressively unresponsive and required intubation and mechanical ventilation.

Prayer 175 (December 5, 2020)
In olden days Lord, when your people were afflicted and they repented and called your name, you mercifully forgave and rescued them.
We have fallen away from you Lord, but a remnant remains that still believes.
We repent and call your holy name. Loving Father hear us.
When we are delivered, those who believe will know who saved us – not the politicians, not the scientists and doctors, but the hand of our almighty Father in Heaven who has dominion in all things above and below! Glory to our loving God!

Donovan's lungs "whited out" – *became completely opaque on the chest X-ray* – indicating they were almost completely full of pus. He was entombed in a proning bed and dialysis was started. I talked with his family and we changed his code status to DNR – Do Not Resuscitate.

Sometime that afternoon, I caught up with my patient care duties and tried to call and report to as many of my patients' families as I could. There were many patients on my list that were inappropriately full code, but I decided to attend to Isabella first – *I owed her.*

"Denise? This is Doctor Eckshar calling from the hospital. I'm one of Isabella's doctors. I'm sorry to call you like this, but I'm afraid I have some bad news about how Isabella is doing.

She's in a tough spot here. She isn't responding to therapy. As you know, she had to go on a ventilator the other day. If she was younger, she would have a better chance, but her age is against her now. She told me the other day that she was tired of the IVs and oxygen. Did your mom ever talk to you about what she would have wanted if she was ever in a situation like this?"

"No, doctor, Mom didn't like talking about serious things like that."

"Hmm. I think I got a little taste of that the other day. You know, I have to share something with you, Denise. I only met your mom about a week and a half ago, but I feel like I know her a little. The day I met her, I was down in the dumps – things are pretty hard here in the ICU right now – and she started joking around with me. I asked her if she wanted anything and she asked for a cold Corona beer! Here I am supposed to be the doctor, but your sick mom cheered me up with her great sense of humor. Anyway, I wanted to tell you, I think your mom is a great lady."

Denise chuckled, "Sounds like mom. Thanks, doctor. Listen, I understand what you need from me. Let me talk with my sister and I'll get back to you. We don't want Mom to suffer." *I didn't want that for Isabella either.*

After we hung up, I looked down my list of 28 Covid patients, all doing badly. How many more spouses, sons, or daughters could I call with such bad news?

Prayer 176 (December 8, 2020)
The Lord is my shepherd I shall not want.
He makes me lie down in green pastures.
He leads me beside quiet waters. He restores my soul.
He guides me in paths of righteousness for his name's sake.
Even though I walk through the valley of the shadow of death, I shall fear no evil, for you are with me.
Your rod and staff comfort me.
You prepare a table for me in the presence of my enemies.
You anoint my head with oil – my cup overflows.

Surely goodness and mercy will follow me all the days of my life, and I will dwell in the house of the Lord forever.

This was one of the toughest days of my life, so I fell back on my old standby prayer: Psalm 23. Multiple personal tragedies struck our family and close friends and the ICU was a nightmare. It was all too much to recount here. I just went from one heartbreak to the next at work. I texted my bible study friends: "Brothers, I'm a little bit at a loss for words at what's happening around me – please pray for the families of all the sick." And received this reply: "Thanks to Jesus, we're never in the valley of death – just shadows. Look to him. Pure light. He restores our souls."

That afternoon, I received a text from Sam, Isabella's nurse of the day: "Daughter and god-daughter of the patient in 372 (Isabella) are here to withdraw life support and transition to comfort care. They wanted to give you a photo of Isabella when she was 40, to see what she looked like before. They felt blessed by your care and sharing the story about how she made you laugh." There was a beautiful smiling picture of Isabella attached, which my drawing below doesn't do justice to. Isabella blessed me when I needed it again. *Godspeed to Jesus's arms my sister!*

Isabella celebrating her birthday with family in 1975.

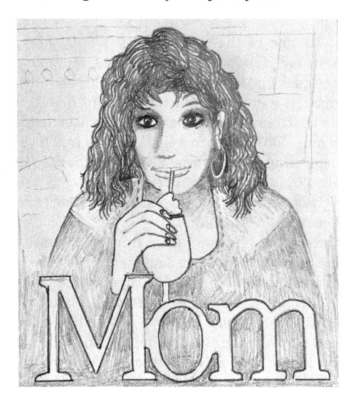

Prayer 177 (December 10, 2020)
*I set the Lord always before me, like a ship sailing by the north star,
for he is at my right hand that I may not be shaken.
Therefore my heart is glad, my tongue rejoices; and my whole body
dwells in hope.
For you will not abandon my soul to hell or let your holy child see
corruption.
You've made known to me the paths of life and you fill me with joy
in your presence!*
[Another prayer based on Psalm 16]

Email:

> To: All Medical and Allied Health Staff
> Date: Wednesday, December 10, 2020
> Subject line: COVID–19 Vaccine update
>
> Colleagues,
> Our healthcare system, in partnership with the Maricopa County Department of Public Health and other community partners, will be offering the COVID–19 vaccine to eligible healthcare workers who desire to receive the vaccine. While we are still awaiting final guidance from the county on the types of healthcare workers that will be eligible, **it is anticipated that those serving on the front lines and with direct patient contact will be given the highest priority for the first dose.**
>
> This week, you will receive an important email with a link to be considered for prioritization of the optional COVID–19 vaccine. These emails have been staggered to accommodate the potentially high volume of interest in case everyone signs up at once.
>
> Once the vaccine is available and the vaccination site is open, you'll receive a message via your cell phone asking you to schedule appointments for your two doses of vaccination **when your priority tier is called.**

An interim analysis of a randomized controlled clinical trial that enrolled 43,500 patients showed that the Pfizer vaccine was >90% effective at preventing Covid infection, with no serious safety concerns. Mass production of the vaccine was being successfully facilitated by President Trump's somewhat goofily-named, but effective "Operation Warp-speed."

I had largely gotten over Covid anxiety. By God's grace and our exhaustive adherence to PPE, most of our team had avoided catching Covid so far, although essentially immersed in it every day. But we now had a new way to protect our family, our friends and ourselves, and I was excited about it.

Frontline medical staff were supposed to be classified "1a" along with ambulance crews and residents of long-term care facilities – the first priority for vaccination. But we had to sign up on a website that scheduled vaccine appointments based on responses to some ambiguous questions. Strangely, although all the doctors and nurses in our unit shared equivalent high-exposure risk, some were allowed to immediately schedule a vaccine appointment, while others were assigned a lower priority and not allowed to schedule. Over the next few days, we all helped each other with the website, double-checking to be sure no one was left behind. It was with a sense of great accomplishment (my computer skills are atrocious) that I helped two nurses truthfully correct their website responses to get them into the first tier where they belonged. Two other nurses decided to hold off on vaccination – both had previously experienced potentially life-threatening anaphylactic vaccine reactions (the most dangerous form of allergy). The rest of us juggled our schedules to get vaccinated as soon as possible. I was able to finagle an appointment for myself on Friday, December 17, just before I was scheduled to go back on duty.

Later that day, Inez, the patient Dom and I had taken care of fifteen years ago, texted me to let me know her father had passed away from Covid. I called her with my condolences and we spent some time catching up. Inez was going to temporarily move in with her mom Marta (who once thought I was a visitation of Jesus) to help her grieve. I told her to let Marta know I was praying for her.

Prayer 178 (December 12, 2020)
The great I am!
You said "Let there be light" and the universe came into being.
Everything that happened since and everything that ever will happen hangs on your word.
Who are we to question you – even to pray to you?

We only can because you made us to love us, and you came down among us as Jesus Christ to redeem us thru the gift of faith.
Protect us Lord.
Sustain us against all earthly turmoil and spiritual attack and use us today to further your kingdom on Earth.

On this dismal day, I arrived at work to learn that three of my Covid pneumonia patients had passed away overnight. But Donovan's oxygenation was improving, and he was supined. I stopped his sedation medications and put his ventilator in a mode that allowed him to start taking partial control of his own breathing again. He was still only minimally responsive, but that was expected. It would probably take him a few days to clear all the sedation drugs he had received. I remembered Donovan's code status was DNR, and I called his family to recommend that we reinstate full code status given he re-emergence of hope. They seemed unusually reserved about what I thought was finally some good news. They only half-heartedly agreed to resume full code status.

Donovan's sister Nora was transferred from the general medicine ward to the ICU and intubated. She had been taken care of by our hospitalists the previous two weeks with a BiPAP mask but had finally exhausted all her reserves.

Prayer 179 (December 14, 2020)
Brace us Lord Jesus against the difficulties of life. Lift us up.
Give us endurance against pain, hope to overcome anxiety, trust that you will never abandon us and faith to know that all things serve your purpose.
Somehow all things ultimately turn out good for those you love.
Prepare us for your kingdom. All glory and praise to you.
[From Ezekiel 11 and 12]

Our census peaked at 45 patients (170% of the maximum safe census), 39 with Covid pneumonia. Somehow, we were able to see all our patients, although this would previously have seemed impossible.

Donovan wasn't waking up as quickly as expected, and at Isaiah's suggestion, I ordered a CT brain scan. The scan showed a large hemorrhagic stroke* in the right frontal lobe that ruptured internally into the ventricles of his brain. I called Donovan's daughter and mom to give them the disastrous news. They seemed unsurprised. I didn't have to convince them it was time to call it quits. Donovan's mom, son and two daughters came in to be with him when we removed the ventilator and let him die.

Down the ICU hallway, Donovan's sister Nora was rapidly deteriorating, now on 80% oxygen and proned, her kidneys shutting down. Two days after Donovan's death, his family refused consent for dialysis and withdrew life support on Nora.

I think they were emotionally compromised by Donovan's death – *as were we all*. I sometimes wonder what might have happened if we had held in there for Nora. But I guess none of us had much gas left in the tank by then.

[*Covid causes a derangement in blood coagulation that increases the chance of stroke by about twenty times during the course of Covid infection.*]

Prayer 180 (December 15, 2020)
Dear Lord, you promised the upright shall behold your face.
I think this means that we will finally become who you meant us to be.
It means dawn will rise on the dark night of this fallen world.
We will finally come home to Eden with you.
We will be with the One of whom even the greatest earthly friendships are only a faint glimpse and to whom the most sublime earthly joys are finally pointing.
[Offered by Mike U. based on Psalm 11 and Revelations 22]

During check-in, Mayfield told me something funny that happened overnight. At about 3 am, he was rounding in the unit when he heard a terrible noise coming from room

318, currently occupied by a 49-year-old Covid patient named Hurley. Unearthly, raucous breath sounds; Hurley must be choking to death! Mayfield mentally compiled a differential diagnosis as he slammed on his PPE: *ETT dislodged? Tube cuff ruptured? Ventilator tubing disconnected?* Fully gowned and masked, he burst into the room to save Hurley's life!

Hurley was still properly connected to the ventilator, and the ETT was in place. Where was that racket coming from? He espied an iPad on Hurley's bedside table displaying the slumbering visage of Hurley's wife, Rita. She had fallen asleep watching over him. The terrible uproar was her snoring, amplified over the iPad speakers!

The nurses later told me that Hurley and Rita had established a routine of spending the nights together by iPad. Although Hurley obviously couldn't speak while intubated, he could listen to Rita, and they could see each other. This helped Hurley sleep without requiring as much sedation.

Prayer 181 (December 17, 2020)
Jesus, you have taught me what righteousness is.
Your law resides in my heart.
I will not forget my maker.
I will not fear the reproach of man, or be dismayed at their revilings.
For they will rot away, but your righteousness is forever, and your salvation to all generations.
You are he who comforts the world.
You stretched out the Heavens and laid the foundations of the Earth.
You stirred up the sea so that its waves roar.
You have put your words in our hearts and covered us in the shadow of your hand.
You alone are the Lord our God – The Lord of Hosts, and you have proclaimed, "You are my people."
[From Isaiah 51]

On December 17, 2020, I received my first dose of the Pfizer

Covid vaccine. I had anticipated this with great excitement. I was scheduled to begin another cluster of shifts over the upcoming weekend and was happy to get the vaccine in my system before my next potential exposure.

Jean kindly drove me to the massive drive-through vaccination site, located in an expansive parking lot. She wasn't eligible to be vaccinated yet, but I was probably her main Covid exposure risk – *my vaccination would protect her too*. We only waited about 15 minutes in a line of cars before pulling up to a tent where I presented my ID, which was checked against my appointment information. Then we were directed by flag-waving volunteers to "lane 6," one of eight mobile vaccine administration tents set up in the parking lot. A few more questions, rolled up my sleeve, a quick jab in the deltoid, a band-aid slapped-on, and I was done. We were supposed to wait in the parking lot for 15 minutes to be sure I didn't have an allergic reaction, but we cut out a few minutes early. Another testament to American ingenuity: effective mass vaccinations were being rolled out <u>less than one year</u> after China announced the emergence of Covid.

Prayer 182 (December 19, 2020)
Let my heart seek you Lord.
Let me see your creative hand in all nature, in the plants and animals, the sunrise, the Milky Way.
Let me see your control over my destiny in all my daily ups and downs – encouragements and opportunities to build my reliance on you. Let me see your spirit in all people.
You made each of us with equal perfection according to your will, and only you can rightly judge who is pleasing in your eyes.
Let me feel your presence around me and in me whenever I make a decision, so that I can remember Jesus: "I only serve one Lord – you."
Let me find peace in your shadow whenever I feel lonely, anxious or depressed and remember none of these make any sense as long as you smile on me.

Our ICU Covid census hovered in the mid-40s. We had 20 deaths from Covid in the ten days leading up to Christmas, five in a single day. Multiple friends in Phoenix, Payson and Chicago had come down with Covid. One of my best friends in Payson was coughing while telling me about his Christmas family dinner plans. I recommended he take a Covid test. This seemed an obvious suggestion, but he was a bit taken aback and it took him a few days to decide whether or not to follow through. His Covid test came back positive on Christmas Eve. Like many other families, their celebration of Christmas 2020 was ruined by Covid.

Inez called me. Nine days after the death of her father from Covid pneumonia, she and her 84-year-old mother Marta both had coughs. I recommended Inez bring Marta in immediately for Covid testing; she was a good candidate for monoclonal antibody treatment. Inez agreed; she said she would take her to the doctor as soon as her mom got home from church.

One of Covid's terrible spiritual/psychological effects was the estrangement of faithful people from their places of worship. This was triggered in March 2020, when a super-spreader event occurred at a Christian choir practice in Washington State; 45 of 60 choir members subsequently contracted Covid and two died. In response, the CDC issued a warning against singing in church. And to many, this seemed an infringement of the First Amendment, which provides that Congress make no law respecting an establishment of religion or prohibiting its free exercise.

I think this led many believers to distrust official public education efforts, disregard the risk of congregating and even deny Covid was a legitimate threat. Some said that God would protect them from Covid. *"I am vaccinated by the blood of Christ" I saw on one lady's T-shirt.* But we have not been promised immunity from disease by Christ's sacrifice. And I don't think the Father wants us to demonstrate our faith by purposely putting ourselves in harm's way. Satan once tried to tempt Jesus that way. Jesus refused and responded, "You shall not put the Lord your God to the test." [Luke 4:12]. Believers like me <u>needed</u> to lean into our faith during the pandemic, but there are ways to worship and exercise faith without putting your friends, family, or self in peril.

Prayer 183 (December 21, 2020)
Through you Lord Jesus, we have obtained access by faith into your Father's grace, in which we stand, and we rejoice in the glory of God!
Not only that, but with your Holy Spirit, we can even rejoice in our sufferings, knowing that in our suffering you bestow endurance, in endurance character, and in character, hope.
And hope in you will never put us to shame, because your love has been poured into our hearts through the gift of your Holy Spirit.
[From Romans 5:1-5]

Our hospital surge plan was fully implemented. The trauma surgeons were taking as many of the non-Covid ICU patients as they could. We appreciated the anesthesiologists and ER docs who helped us out on some of our worst days, but they were out of their element, and it was difficult to effectively work them into our workflow. Behind the scenes, our most important physician support came from the hospitalists. As bad as our ICU census was, it would have been much worse except for these hard-working and resourceful physicians.

Hospitalists are internal medicine physicians specializing in hospital work; they do the "grunt work" when specialists admit patients. During the pandemic, hospitalists quietly raised the threshold for ICU transfer. I was repeatedly amazed by floor patients transferred to the ICU who were sick enough to be in the unit weeks earlier. It turns out that dozens of such patients were properly cared for on the floor with BiPAP masks and high-flow nasal oxygen, not because of any explicit administrative surge plan, but simply because the intrepid hospitalists were individually all stepping up to hold the line, only transferring patients who *absolutely* needed the

ICU. Thereby saving our bacon. My thanks go out to all the hospitalists who held the line for us.

Prayer 184 (December 25, 2020, a Christmas prayer)
Great and wise Father, how good it is that Christmas is at the end of our year. We had a tough one Father.
We brought great disaster on ourselves.
We largely turned away from you,
as we have so many other times in the past.
You would be entirely righteous to abandon us if not for the blood of your Son.
But here we are, having survived 2020 because of your mercy and loving-kindness, the forgiveness that Christ earned for us, and the gifts of faith and the Holy Spirit.
And now we are in remembrance of the second greatest day in history, the day you sent your holy perfect Son down into the dirt to be one of us and save us.
Kind Father and loving Son – we remember what you did for us when we were filthy and hostile.
How much more will you bless us in 2021, having been made clean by Christ and having had our faith strengthened by you through the adversity we suffered together last year.
2021 is coming – Let it be the year of the Lord's mercy!

Despite this prayer, I had little abiding Christmas spirit and no sense of celebration. Work and recovering from work were all-encompassing, leaving no mental energy for anything else.

One of the twenty-odd patients I saw at work today, Rachel, was a 46-year-old Hopi woman with Covid pneumonia who had been intubated five days. She spiked a 102-degree fever and ETT cultures revealed *Klebsiella pneumoniae* bacteria that was "pan-sensitive" – almost any reasonable antibiotic I might pick was likely to be effective, *at least theoretically*. I started her on a single strong IV antibiotic, ceftriaxone, for ten days. My impression – *that should do the trick* – would later be disastrously disproven.

When I got home from work, Jean had made a nice dinner for us, but I was too tired to do much more than wolf it down. I had given up living in the guest room months ago, and I went upstairs to our bedroom, flopped face-down in bed – *proned you might say* – on top of the blankets, fully dressed, without even taking my shoes off, and passed out.

Prayer 185 (December 26, 2020)
The day after Christmas sometimes feels like a letdown.
But Lord, you lift us up daily.
Let us never forget that your incarnation leads to an ultimate joy for all of us, even through pain and suffering, loss and disappointment, anxiety and confusion.
Please let the hope of this joy carry us into this New Year.
Please let all of those who have lost loved ones come to know you and ultimately their tears will be wiped away.
Thank you for the gift of your Son, and may our hearts now stay filled with Christmas joy.
Please give us the strength to carry that joy to others and to love our fellow man the way you showed. In Jesus' holy name we pray.
[from Mike U.]

I saw 28 critically ill patients on my shift – the most patients I had ever seen in my career – single-handedly exceeding what we had previously determined as the maximum safe census for *two* ICU docs.

Hurley had now been in the ICU for 21 days, proned on 90% oxygen with sky-high ventilator pressures, his kidneys failing. His wife Rita continued to spend each night with him by video, but Hurley was comatose now. He suffered secondary bacterial pneumonia with antibiotic-resistant *Staphylococcus aureus*, and he was spiking fevers of 103 degrees. Two days later, his right lung ruptured and his sputum culture grew an antibiotic-resistant bacteria called *Pseudomonas aeruginosa*.

It was time. Again. I knew I should call Rita and recommend comfort care. But I couldn't. Maybe I was just too exhausted by all the death; maybe the iPad story made Hurley's care too personal to me. Whatever the reason, I ordered a second course of dexamethasone – increasing the dose about ten times. I asked Alvarez, one of our nephrologists, to start dialysis, worried he might deride me for further torturing Hurley in what seemed a futile situation. But if Alvarez felt that way, at least he didn't let his feelings show. He wrote the orders. Dialysis might give Hurley a few more days to see if the steroids would work.

Prayer 186 (December 27, 2020)
O Lord, you have laid your hand upon me.
You know when I lie down and when I rise.
My mind is an open book to you and not a word leaves my tongue before you know it.
You are all about my path, fashioning my past, present and future.
You placed me in my mother's womb.
I thank you, for I am fearfully and wonderfully made –
How I love your Holy Spirit in me!
How great are your councils and blessings – numbering like the grains of sand in all the world.
Try me Lord. Seek the ground of my heart.
Prove me and examine my thoughts.
Look well, take any wickedness from me and lead me in your everlasting presence. [Adaptation of Psalm 139]

Hurley's dialysis had not yet been started. The skin around his neck and chest was filled with crepitant air from his ruptured lung. This obscured the ultrasound images of the underlying veins used to guide dialysis IV placement by the line technician. There was no safe way for the technician to place the line: no line, no dialysis.

Back in the day before ultrasound machines, we used to place dialysis lines "blindly" using a little knowledge of vascular anatomy and a lot of experience earned through trial and error. I hadn't placed a deep central dialysis catheter without ultrasound guidance for over a decade but had

previously done hundreds. I was pretty sure I could still do it –
Lord, don't let me be wrong.

I asked the line team to "assist me"(essentially to do almost
the entire procedure except for the critical first step: finding
the femoral vein deep in Hurley's groin by touch alone,
needling it and placing a steel guidewire into it). Once we were
all gowned and gloved and Hurley was prepped, my part took
no more than five minutes and went smooth as silk. *The hands
have a long memory.* I pressed the pads of my left fingers into
the crease of the groin – presser deeper until I could feel the
femoral pulse. Then plunged the nearly four-inch-long needle
into the groin, about a half centimeter medially, where my
fingers thought the femoral vein must lie, applying syringe
suction continuously. *The vein should be right about . . . there!*
The syringe suddenly filled with dark venous blood. I carefully
held the needle in place, popped the syringe off and passed
the steel guidewire about 20 cm through the needle and into
the vein, then pulled the needle out over the wire. The dialysis
catheter could be passed over this guidewire into the vein.
Although I think I looked outwardly impassive, I was pretty
nervous and had been silently praying before, during and after.
"Can you guys take it from here?"

"You're done already!?"

"Yes. Thank God!" I suppressed a smile, could tell the
line techs were impressed. Those old-timers who have done
this simple blind procedure would laugh at the thought
I'm bragging about it. What would have been an expected
competency for an intern in 1986 seemed magical to the line
technicians in 2021. Ultrasound technology made deep IV line
placement safer and easier, but it was nice to know that *just
once in a blue moon*, the old ways still had value. Hurley's
dialysis got started later that afternoon.

Prayer 187 (December 31, 2020)
Father God. You carried us through a tough year in 2020.
We would never have survived it without your mercy, your gift of

faith, and the love for each other you put in our hearts.
We don't know what 2021 has in store for us, but we know that we
are under your protection Lord, now and in the future.
Nothing can separate us from your love.

Our hospital was a neurology specialty center, typically staffed by four inpatient neurologists. But right at the onset of the pandemic, two of our neurologists abruptly quit.

Dr. Richards, one of the pair that stuck with us, was in his early 70s, tireless, kind and humorous. He accepted the risk of Covid exposure and extra workload without complaint. As he later told me, he subsequently took call for neurology emergencies at the hospital continuously, 24 hours a day, seven days a week, from March thru November 2020. "I did what anyone would do." *No, Richards, you did what only you would do!*

Richards seemed to have near-photographic memory. A typical statement from him regarding a consult went something like this: "The patient has anti-Hu antibody paraneoplastic cerebral ataxia due to spindle cell cancer. Treatment of choice according to the British Medical Journal, 2015, volume 15, page 998: chemotherapy of the primary tumor." If that was over your head, join the club. Everyone acknowledged Richards was the smartest doc around.

On this day, a grinning Dr. Richards came driving down the hallway of the ICU on the hospital floor-scrubbing machine. He had convinced one of our good-hearted housecleaners into loaning him the keys to what we all called "the Zamboni" and did several laps around the ICU, waving from his perch like a parade queen, to the delight and muted cheers of the nurses and doctors. A crazy sight – *a sign perhaps we were all losing it* – Richards lightened the mood and gave us a laugh we needed on that dismal holiday

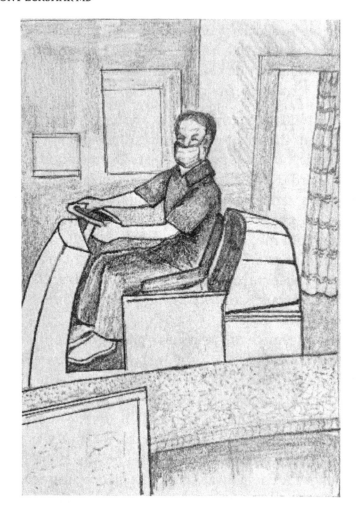

Prayer 188 (January 4, 2021)
Lord, In the quiet of the night, let my mind be at peace.
Let my body rest easy and my sleep be untroubled.
For you are my protector – the one who stays vigilant and defends
me from all adversity.
There is no enemy that can overcome you, my shepherd! My Lord!
I trust in you and therefore I will not fear.

Prayer 189 (January 6, 2021)
Heavenly Father, we remember long ago, how you spared a people
from destruction for the sake of a remnant who were righteous. We

are not righteous on our own account Lord, but by the blood of your Son!
We have rejected you as a nation more than ever these past years. But the remnant of your people cry out to you in the name of Christ: "Father, spare our country for your name's sake!"
Help us rebuild our country to be how we thought it was supposed to be when we said the pledge of allegiance as kids – "One nation under God, indivisible, with liberty and justice for all."

Arizona once again achieved the highest per capita rate of Covid infection of any region in the world, based on data published by Johns Hopkins University. A person was dying from Covid every 10-15 minutes in Arizona. Yet surreally, we didn't have a state facemask mandate, and schools, gyms, restaurants and nightclubs were open for business as usual. Many people who didn't work in healthcare were apparently entirely unaware of the carnage unfolding in hospitals all over the city.

Meanwhile, on the seventeenth day of her hospitalization, and only one day after her course of ceftriaxone antibiotic was completed, Rachel spiked another high fever. This time, her ETT cultures grew a Klebsiella bacteria with intermediate resistance to multiple antibiotics. A cocktail of some of our strongest antibiotics was started. As Rachel continued to slowly worsen over the next three weeks, various combinations of five different antibiotics were tried without success in an effort to eradicate this organism.

Prayer 190 (January 8, 2020)
Many of my friends are now sick with Covid.
Several have lost their parents and other close relatives.
We are beat-down Lord and losing hope in earthly authorities, but as worldly adversity increases, your mercy and love increase even more.
You have brought us all closer together so that we would help each other.

You have given us each our role to play in duty and love.
Great Father, we lean on you more than ever.
You are our rock and our salvation.
A broken spirit and a contrite heart you will not despise.
Carry us through Lord; do not let us fall.

I was in the hospital cafeteria, mechanically chewing my breakfast while anxiously contemplating my worklist – *it didn't look good* – when I became aware that something wasn't quite right. I felt a little light-headed, and I could sense a rapid palpitation behind my breastbone. I checked my radial pulse – *very fast* – 150 beats per minute. I never had anything like this before. *It should pass in minute.* I set my coffee aside, took a few deep breaths, and tried to relax . . . *It didn't pass.* Not sure what else to do, I took the stairs up to the unit, one at a time, tracked down our EKG tech, and asked them to wire me up for an informal study. The EKG revealed atrial flutter. There wasn't much I could do about it that wouldn't significantly interrupt my workday. I felt good enough to work. I started seeing patients and about an hour later, noticed my heart rate had popped back into normal rhythm.

Hurley was improving; down to 40% oxygen, coming off sedation, and his kidney function recovering. I considered how close I came to giving up on him with some uneasiness. Four days later, he was extubated and was rapidly recovering strength with the help of our physical therapists. I found out later that Hurley and his wife, Rita, were separated before his illness. I don't know whether they got back together or not, but Hurley's wife surely demonstrated a great deal of love throughout their ordeal together. That should count for something.

I checked in with Inez – she and her mom had both tested positive for Covid, but were feeling better already, thank God.

Prayer 191 (January 11, 2021)
Thank you Lord Jesus.

The parting of the Red Sea is no more difficult for you than this.
Some prayer miracles are great and some are small.
Either way, we recognize the work of your mighty hands
for those you love.
Open our eyes Lord to all your myriad acts of kindness, mercy and love in our lives! We praise your holy name!

On January 11, 2021, The Covid surge finally peaked in Arizona, with 5082 Covid patients occupying hospital beds, 1183 in ICUs and 786 on ventilators. There were 390 Covid deaths in Arizona the following day – a Covid death every four minutes!

Prayer 192 (January 16, 2021)
Lord we are broken-hearted and exhausted.
We need you now more than ever.
Do not turn your face away from us– your lost sheep, afraid in the wilderness.
Do not let us be put to shame for our trust in you.
We do trust you, merciful and kind Father!
Lift up our heads!
Put your mighty hand on our brother's head and heal him as you did those who cried out to Jesus.
Don't withhold your healing power from us now Lord.
Your will be done. Let your name be glorified!

In mid-January, one of my old colleagues and friends, Dr. Hamlet Lee, spiked a fever the day after receiving his first Covid vaccine shot. This initially seemed merely a side effect, but when he started coughing and became short of breath a few days later, he knew something was up. Lee – *"Ham" just never seemed an appropriate nickname* – was diagnosed with Covid pneumonia and admitted to a neighboring hospital. As the horrific events of the next few months unfolded, I wondered many times how things might have been different if he had only received his vaccination a week or two earlier.

I have to tell a quick background story about Lee. He

was one of my favorite attendings at the hospital I trained-in back in the mid-1980s. I was a lowly intern and Lee was a successful and highly respected specialist. A certain social barrier generally maintained a distance between the two, but not so between us. Whenever we worked together, Lee always set me at ease and treated me as a colleague. One way he had of doing this was by telling jokes. My favorite was a true personal story he once shared with me.

Lee said he once entered an exam room to see a female patient who had a curious chief complaint. Lee was wearing his stethoscope hanging off his neck by the curved stainless steel ear tubes – a common way doctors tote their stethoscope around. He was distracted thinking about her differential diagnosis as he moved in close to examine her and forgot to put the earpieces in his ears before placing the bell of his stethoscope over her heart. Of course, to his momentary consternation, he couldn't hear a thing. The patient immediately noticed his blunder and remarked, "Aren't those ear things supposed to be in your ears?" *It seemed like something I would have done, not Lee!*

There never was a more professional physician than Lee by any prevailing definition. That's why his humane sharing of this embarrassing story with a lowly intern meant so much to me. He was human despite the suit. By sharing this story he reminded me that neither of us was anything fancy. When you came right down to it, we were basically still just two guys with stethoscopes.

Prayer 193 (January 18, 2021, Martin Luther King Day)
God grant that right here in America and all over this world,
we will choose the high way; a way in which men will live together as brothers.
A way in which the nations of the world will beat their swords into plowshares, and their spears into pruning hooks.
A way in which every man will respect the dignity and worth of all human personality.

A way in which every nation will allow justice to run down like waters, and righteousness like a mighty stream.

A way in which men will do justly, love mercy, and walk humbly with God.

A way in which men will be able to stand up, and in the midst of oppression, in the midst of darkness and agony, they will be able to stand there and love their enemies, bless those persons that curse them, pray for those individuals that despitefully use them.

And this is the way that will bring us once more into that society which we think of as the brotherhood of man.

This will be that day when white people, colored people, whether they are brown or whether they are yellow or whether they are black, will join together and stretch out with their arms and be able to cry out: "Free at last! Free at last! Great God Almighty, we are free at last!" [Dr. Martin Luther King Jr.]

Hurley was transferred out of the ICU to a skilled nursing facility, eventually recovering and returning home. I liked to hope he and Rita patched things up.

Prayer 194 (January 19, 2021)

Be merciful to me God, for in you my soul takes refuge; in the shadow of your wings shall I rest until the storms of destruction pass by.

My soul is in the midst of lions, but my heart is steadfast for I trust in you.

O God, I will give thanks to you!

O Lord, I will sing praises to you, for your steadfast love is as great as the Heavens; your faithfulness reaches above the clouds.

Be exalted God – let your glory reign over all the Earth!

[Psalm 57 abbreviated]

I admitted Dallas, a 52-year-old man with chronic psychiatric illness, made homeless three months earlier by the death of his mother. He was febrile and short of breath for about a week before seeking medical attention. He required

100% oxygen through a BiPAP mask in the ER to keep his O2 sats above 90% and I was shocked by the degree of respiratory distress he was in when he arrived in the ICU. He had waited until the last possible moment to seek aid. With BiPAP support, he was breathing ten times more air than a normal person would,* requiring an incredible respiratory effort that couldn't possibly be maintained. As I prepared as quickly as possible to intubate him, Dallas went into respiratory arrest.

Dallas coded three times over the next hour. Each time we got a pulse back, his blood pressure immediately started drifting down until it was lost again. I performed an echocardiogram of his heart during his third brief recovery. The right side of his heart was massively dilated and a huge blood clot could be seen in his right atrium – it was hung up there somehow, prolapsing back and forth across the tricuspid heart valve, threatening to break free and travel to his lungs with every feeble heartbeat. [*Such blood clots in the legs, heart and lungs were found to be increased 5-10 times in patients with Covid due to the complex detrimental effects the virus has on blood coagulation.*] I administered a bolus of the clot-busting medication "tPA," and Dallas's blood pressure firmly stabilized shortly thereafter.

Ninety minutes had gone by since Dallas had arrived in the unit. The code team was spent. The room looked like a bomb had gone off – the bedsheets twisted and soiled with blood and respiratory secretions, IV lines tangled with oximeter cords and EKG monitoring leads, empty ACLS drug ampules and packaging from the central IV line kit and intubation equipment littering the floor. Ultimately, it was all for nothing. Dallas survived the day but never regained consciousness and passed away before the end of the week.

[*A normal person breathes about a half liter of air twelve times per minute (0.5L x 12 breaths/minute = 6L/minute). Dallas was breathing one and a half liters of air forty times per minute (1.5 x 40 = 60L/minute.*]

Prayer 195 (January 20, 2021)
Oh God, you know my failings; the wrongs I have done are not hidden from you.
Let not those who hope in you be put to shame through me.
Let not those who seek you be brought to dishonor through me.
If I must bear reproach, let it be for your sake rather than for my failings.
Let zeal for your house consume me, even if I become estranged from my brothers.
But as for me, my prayer is to you!
O Lord, at an acceptable time, in the abundance of your steadfast love, answer me in your saving faithfulness.
Deliver me from the deep waters.
Don't let the flood sweep over me or the deep swallow me up.
Hide not your face from your servant.
Draw near to my soul and redeem me! [Adaptation of Psalm 69]

Lee's condition perilously declined. Although he had only been sick just over a week, he already required 80% oxygen by BiPAP mask. Over the next 48 hours, he was intubated and required 100% oxygen.

Prayer 196 (January 21, 2021)
I remember the story you once told about the unjust judge who gave a woman petitioner the justice she sought only because of her persistence.
How much more, merciful Father, will you hear the petitions of your children for Lee – a man who you love?
We are not going to stop pestering you until you grant our prayer, because we have faith in you!
Heal Lee and all who suffer from Covid, Lord for your glory.

I had a few days off from the ICU, and our drive-through Covid vaccination site needed workers. Volunteers were eligible to receive thawed unused vaccine doses, which would otherwise be wasted at the end of the day. I felt great to be able to get this protection for Jean and do something proactive in the fight against Covid. Jean and I signed up to work on January 20th. Jean was assigned to the information/communication team organizing the event, and I was assigned to administer vaccine shots.

I staffed one of eight vaccination tents at the site, along with two retired docs, an anesthesiologist and an obstetrician. Although we had well over a century of cumulative medical experience between us, none of us had ever administered a vaccine shot before – a task usually assigned to nurses. The positive nature of what we were doing and the absurdity of our lack of such a simple job skill put us all in good humor as we reviewed what we had learned in the training videos.

As each car pulled up, we asked them to turn off their engine, asked their name and date of birth, pulled them up on the computer and verified their appointment and eligibility criteria. Vaccine syringes were pre-thawed and kept in a cooler in the shade. We took turns instructing each patient to stick their arm out the car window, sleeve rolled-up above the shoulder. When it was my turn to give a jab, I swiped the skin over the deltoid with an alcohol wipe, pinched the skin, jabbed the needle squeezing the plunger quickly, then pulled out and slapped a band-aid on. It was my philosophy that the less time a patient had to think about it, the less it would hurt. The needles were so small and sharp that most patients didn't feel a thing – a seemingly minor victory that I took a disproportionate degree of pride in. Someone had the cute idea of handing out Dum-Dums lollipops to each vaccinated person like we got after a shot when we were kids. We let each person select their favorite flavor from a Costco-sized variety pack.

Two of our victims were police officers in a marked Phoenix PD Ford Explorer. When they drove up, I asked them to pull over, roll their window down and turn their motor off. Then I asked them if they knew why I had pulled them over. They chuckled. "I've been waiting my whole life to say that to some cops."

Another customer was a 98-year-old man whose daughter had chauffeured him to the site. I addressed the gentleman with a straight face, "Sorry sir, we are only vaccinating people over 100 today – you'll have to come back in 2 years." They cracked up.

I had more fun giving vaccine shots that day. I couldn't remember feeling this way – just doing a simple job that I couldn't fail at, a job that made a positive difference. It felt like we were putting Covid behind us. I have to admit, I felt greater job satisfaction volunteering at the vaccination site than I had for the past nine months in the ICU.

Prayer 197 (January 23, 2021)
God, every day our hopes go up or down – all over the place.
We don't know whether to rejoice or despair.
But your will and your plan do not waver.
They are rock solid and for sure.
If you say Lee is going to get well, it doesn't matter what his oxygen level is, or what his chest X-ray looks like.
Your word is law, so we will not despair! We have faith in you, and we know our faith will not go unnoticed, merciful Father.
Hear our cry! Say the word and it will be so.

Lee's first week in the hospital followed the same trajectory as many of our sickest Covid patients. He was now on near-maximal ventilator support providing 100% oxygen. I cared about every one of my patients, but witnessing one of my personal friends and his family getting washed away down this deadly river hit my soul from a different angle. Maybe it was inevitable – by this point, there weren't many people left who couldn't tell a story of how Covid threatened the life of a family member or close friend. I got together with Lee's wife, Daisy, my old partner Jan O'Neill (another of Lee's ex-students) and a few other mutual friends, and we began praying together for Lee by text every day, including Lee in the texts although he wouldn't be able to reply anytime soon.

Prayer 198 (January 24, 2021)

Jesus, you once pointed out that even human parents give good things to their children when they ask for help.

How much more can we trust you, our heavenly Father, to give us any good thing we ask for in faith?

We are asking.

Heal our brothers and sisters from Covid Father.

Heal Lee.

Give them back to us. Don't delay any longer.

Send us an encouraging sign, for the sake of your glory and our faith.

Prayer 199 (January 25, 2021)

The Lord rules.

We praise you and thank you.

Nothing that happens is a coincidence.

Everything happens according to your will and has a purpose in your plan.

You got Lee through today Lord – bless your holy name.

Now, please get him through tomorrow!

We love you Lord. We trust you.

When we are in trouble, we run to you, and you save and protect us.

You will not let us be put to shame for depending on you!

We had forty patients on our ICU service. Thirty-seven had life-threatening Covid pneumonia. But the rate of new Covid admissions seemed to be leveling off.

Mayfield checked out to me this morning. He spent the last two hours of his night shift coding a patient with a ruptured abdominal aortic aneurysm. His patient was hanging onto life by a thread. Mayfield admitted, "I'm so tired, I was almost disappointed he survived the code because you know he's never going home, and it's just more work for us and more suffering for him this way." That sounded cold, but I agreed with Mayfield, and he was 100% right: the patient died six hours later, as he predicted, despite full life support. Mayfield had expressed what I felt about taking care of Dallas. Maybe we were both burning out. My old mentor, Dom Novak, warned me that might happen one day.

My phone pinged. An incoming text: "Sometimes we think if God doesn't immediately respond to our prayer (or not in the way we prefer), he must not be listening or mustn't care. But scripture affirms the opposite: He is listening (Jeremiah 29:12), he does care (1 Peter 5:7), and he's got you (Isaiah 41:10). Trust in prayer today." The incredible timeliness of such messages from my friends was becoming an affirmation of faith for me. You never know God's purpose when you text encouragement to a friend.

Prayer 200 (January 27, 2021)
Father God, you carried me through another tough day in the ICU. We would never have survived it without your mercy, your gift of faith, and the love for each other you put in our hearts.
We don't know what tomorrow has in store for us, but we know that we are under your protection Lord, now and in the future, and nothing can separate us from your love.

I was still thinking about what Mayfield said the day before and contemplating whether or not we were both burning out. I remember witnessing the beginning of the end of Dom's career from burnout in 2008.

We were taking care of a woman named Majorie, a 38-year-old who had undergone a biopsy resection of a liver mass. The pathology of the lesion was benign, but the blood vessels to her liver must have been inadvertently injured during the surgery. She lapsed into a coma from fulminant liver failure post-op and was transferred to the ICU. Dom and I were on service together when Majorie's husband and 8-year-old daughter came in to hear the catastrophic news – *Majorie was almost certainly going to die.*

We met them in the hallway in the middle of the ICU.

Dom introduced us, "Thanks for coming in today." We both shook hands with Majorie's husband and daughter, her little hand limp and cool. "We're Majorie's ICU doctors. She was transferred down to the ICU because there's been a serious complication." Tom looked uncertainly at the little girl, then back to her dad – "I have no easy way to tell you what I have to tell you."

Majorie's husband nodded his head, indicating that Dom could proceed, "It's OK – go ahead."

"Majorie's liver was accidentally injured in the surgery, and well, it has stopped working." Dom paused a moment. "This is very serious. When the liver fails like this, it causes the brain to swell. That's why, when you see Majorie, she won't be able to talk to you." He glanced at the little girl. "Your mom looks asleep, but she won't be able to wake up. We had to put her on the breathing machine to give her oxygen." Dom studied the little girl for a moment – *how could she possibly understand what he was saying?* "We are trying to get a liver transplant for her ..."

The little girl interrupted, "Is mommy going to die without a new liver?"

Tom looked stricken, "Yes – Yes, I'm sorry ..."

Little girl, "Then you can take *my* liver and give it to mommy!"

Dom fell silent. Then a tremor went through him and he turned away – *he had a daughter of his own.* Suddenly I noticed the nurses were all staring at him. He hid his face in his hands and started sobbing. He broke down right in front of everyone. It's hard for anyone who didn't know Dom to realize how shocking this was. Everyone knew he cared deeply for his patients, but he hid it behind a concrete-hard shell of brisk competency and humor. He was like an Ironman at work, the last one you would ever expect to break down.

Dom walked away quickly, out of the unit and down the hall, swiping at his eyes. I stayed behind and finished up a little with Marjorie's family. This event, and many others over a thirty-year span, were cumulatively injuring the empathetic, self-critical Dr Novak from within and would ultimately burn him out. Dom later warned me not to follow him down this path, but what could I do to avoid it?

Prayer 201 (January 28, 2021)
I love how you work Lord.
So far above us in knowledge and in power, yet merciful and loving, answering our prayers in ways we couldn't have imagined.
Though there is nothing you need *us to do to fulfill your will,* but you let us play our parts in your plan to build our faith.
Everything you do to us, for us is an expression of your wisdom and love.
We praise and thank you.
You have brought us to the final stretch of the ICU.
Lord, now please wake Lee up and get him home!

I was fighting hopelessness at this point and did some math to try to wrap my head around why. I looked back to my patient list from a month earlier: on December 28[th,] we saw 33 Covid pneumonia patients. I tracked down what happened to each one now, a month later: 26 were dead, and five were still on ventilators. Only two were extubated and discharged: Hurley and an 82-year-old woman had been discharged to hospice care to die.

All the combined work of our ICU team over the entire month came down to saving only Hurley, who was by no means guaranteed to make it home. It was worth a month of work to save Hurley – but it dawned on me that for all the other 27 patients, the only help I provided was to have prayed for them, perhaps comforting them a little in their final days. Whether that counted for anything was not a question of *this* world.

Prayer 202 (January 29, 2021)
In the Old Testament, the New Testament, and today in our everyday life, God, you reveal yourself to those who have received

your gift of faith.
We have faith Lord – thanks to you.
We put our faith in you, and we know, you never put faith to shame.
We have faith you are going to heal Lee.
You're going to take him off the vent and get him home.
Just say the word Lord. Your word is law on Heaven and Earth.
We come before you. We bow down at your feet.
Hear and answer our prayer.
We only have faith in you!

I was temporarily discouraged by the material futility of the past month's efforts, but not for long. It was too busy to think about much else besides whatever my next task was. We can only each do our duty to the best of our ability. Beyond that, we ought neither to take too much credit for good outcomes nor fault for bad ones. It's all in God's hands.

Lee was making no progress despite the best medical care and daily prayer with Daisy and the circle of Lee's friends. It seemed like he would almost certainly die, and a disquieting question dawned on me. If we continued praying for complete healing for Lee even as that became more and more unlikely, what would happen to our faith when Lee died? *Were we setting ourselves up to be disappointed in God?* This made me briefly wonder if we should instead start praying for strength to submit to God's will rather than for what we really wanted.

But sometime around late January, I decided to keep asking Jesus for complete healing as people did in the Bible, without reserve, for the entirety of my desire, no matter how unlikely it seemed – *after all, how likely was it that a blind man would have his sight restored?* From here on out, we all implicitly agreed to pretend we didn't know how bad things were looking for Lee and to pray for nothing less than his full recovery.

January 30, 2021. Dawn in Payson Arizona - fresh snow overnight. Our 10-year-old Golden Retriever "Jem" running around in deep snow with total abandon.

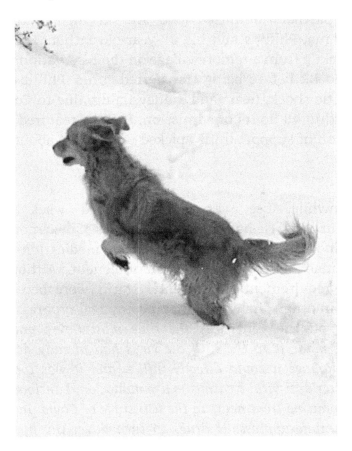

Prayer 203 (January 30, 2021)
People used to sneak up behind you Jesus and just touch the hem of your robe to be cured of incurable diseases.
Some guys once tore a hole in the roof of a house you were in, to lower their crippled friend down by ropes into your presence to be cured.
We bring Lee before you lord Jesus, with hearts like these people had. We bow down to you.

We know we don't have a chance without you, but we are totally confident in your power.
We kneel before you and beg you to heal Lee.

My partners admitted two Navajo men with Covid pneumonia, Phillips and his 87-year-old father. They drove their pickup from a remote village on the reservation to Little Colorado ER before being transferred to us. Phillips' father had septic shock, heart and kidney failure due to Covid and died within 48 hours of admission. Phillips required gradual escalation of support until I picked up his care about a week later.

Meanwhile, Lee was in his second week of ICU hospitalization. He had completed courses of dexamethasone, and another immune-suppressing medication called tocilizumab*, but without apparent benefit. Although his oxygen requirements and mental status were better some days than others, he wasn't making any real progress toward coming off the vent. [*By the time most Covid pneumonia patients made it to the ICU, the virus had already done most of the damage it could directly inflict, and it was too late to administer anti-viral treatments like monoclonal antibodies. The most promising treatments in the ICU stage of Covid pneumonia were immunosuppressant drugs to turn down the hyperactive immune response to Covid, which did more harm than good in such patients.]

Prayer 204 (February 1, 2021)
This year, I often prayed Psalm 23 when I was afraid and I thought about why the metaphor of the good shepherd speaks to our hearts.

Lord, when hard times like these come, we don't know which way to go – we don't have any ability to defend ourselves from the dangers we are facing.

But we have you as our shepherd to help us make the right decisions, to provide for us, and to protect us from all evil.
You even provided us with righteousness, through Jesus's sacrifice.
Lead us safely out of this valley of the shadow of death.
It's only the valley of the shadow of death after all, because you delivered us from death and we are confident that you have abundant life in store for us!

Rachel was now on the 44th day of her hospitalization. She continued to intermittently spike fevers and her ETT cultures were persistently positive despite having received 34 days of coverage with six different antibiotics. Today, her ETT cultures grew a highly resistant *Klebsiella pneumoniae* – a far cry from the pan-sensitive Klebsiella that grew over a month ago. This Klebsiella had acquired resistance to almost all modern antibiotics. The culture also grew a bacteria none of us had ever heard of before called *Achromobacter xylosoxidans*, which was also highly resistant to antibiotics. We consulted infectious disease, and they started a cutting-edge antibiotic combination of ceftazidime/avibactam, only recently available because of an FDA-supported research program to develop a treatment for superbugs like the ones Rachel was now infected with.

Rachel died four days later, having received 38 days of antibiotics without ever having cleared the bacteria in her lungs. It should be noted that she would never have been infected by them if she hadn't first suffered critical lung damage due to Covid in the first place. I considered this akin to a patient dying from sepsis related to a gunshot wound – *the bullet is still the primary cause of death.*

Antibiotic stewardship is the principle good doctors practice of limiting the use of antibiotics to reduce the emergence of bacterial resistance. The ID doc that saw Rachel scolded us for all the antibiotics she received along the way. But practicing antibiotic stewardship under these life-and-death situations can also lead to disaster, as I was soon to experience firsthand.

[*Bacteria sometimes attain resistance when exposed to antibiotics. One of the ways they do this is by sharing mobile resistance genes using an intermediary called a plasmid. Plasmids are similar to viruses except that they "infect" bacteria. In relation to antibiotic resistance, plasmids can contain DNA that encodes enzymes that digest specific antibiotics! A bacterium infected by such a plasmid gains antibiotic resistance, and if the antibiotic is being given to the patient at the time, it conveys a competitive advantage – the resistant bacteria take over. In Rachel's case, multiple such gene transfers would have had to occur to create the multidrug-resistant superbugs she ended up with.]

Prayer 205 (February 3, 2021)
Lord, we know being with you in Heaven will be far better, but we still love the beautiful earthly lives you blessed us with.
We love being together here, no matter how hard we have to struggle.
Please give us more good life together with Lee.
Grant Lee more dinners at home with Daisy, more long talks with his sons, more vacations with his grandkids, more patients for him to see, more students for him to teach.
Please say the word Lord and let your will be done.
Heal Lee completely!

It was clear that Lee wasn't coming off the ventilator any time soon – his oxygen requirements had improved a little but were now stubbornly hovering in the 60-80% range. Although his sedation drugs had been discontinued, he wasn't waking up. A tracheostomy was planned, digging in for a long fight, although none of us would have ever guessed *how* long at the time.

Over the next two days, Mayfield and I filled out 16 death certificates – all but three deaths were primarily due to Covid.

It was rumored that Covid deaths were being exaggerated and that other diagnoses, such as hypertension and diabetes, were the actual cause of many "so-called Covid deaths." I have to speak to that from firsthand experience. Covid patients dying in our ICU *were dying from <u>Covid pneumonia</u> and it's direct complications.* Pneumonia is not caused by hypertension or diabetes, so the true cause of death in these cases could not have been confused. Covid was well-known to cause strokes and pulmonary emboli, so patients such as Dallas and Donovan, who died from blood clot complications of Covid (while receiving life support for Covid pneumonia) also had Covid listed as the primary cause of death. We saw very few patients in our ICU with "incidental Covid" until much later in the pandemic. If there was any incentive for blaming Covid for a non-Covid death, I was never aware of it, and it certainly wouldn't have altered my entries on the many Covid death certificates I completed.

The lethality of Covid overshadowed so much of what we did in the unit every day, that it was hard at the time to realize that our patients died from anything else. This experience during a surge was so profoundly impactful, that I had to review our statistics to convince myself that other fatal diseases, such as cancer, had not somehow taken a vacation during the pandemic.

Prayer 206 (February 4, 2021)
All the daily ups and downs, all the changing lab values, are of no concern to you Lord.
Nothing that happens on Earth can stop your will from coming to fulfillment.
We can be patient Lord.
But we won't stop begging you to hear our prayer.
Whatever your timing – sooner or later – Lord heal Lee and get him home to Daisy!
Surely God, you are with us!
We couldn't make it through one day without you.
Here we are, almost a month into Lee and Daisy's fight with Covid, and we are still standing, by your grace and power and authority.

Thanks for getting us this far Lord.
Now please finish your healing miracle!

Lee underwent a tracheostomy on this day, but his laboratory showed the beginnings of kidney failure.

Prayer 207 (February 9, 2021)
Lord, you raise the humble up.
You put the last first. You soothe the broken-hearted.
You reward faith. You appear to those who seek you.
All glory and praise to you loving Father!

Joyce reported during check-in that Philips was the only conscious patient on our service. He had been in the hospital for eleven days and seemed to be hanging in there, perhaps even getting a little better. I tried to see all the sickest patients first, saving Phillips until midday to have something to look forward to. Phillips and his father had both been admitted to our ICU together, but Phillips had asked the ICU staff not to tell him what happened to his father. He told Joyce he just couldn't take it right now if he found out his father had died. Unfortunately, Phillips' feelings in this matter were prescient –his father had passed away the previous week from Covid cardiomyopathy (heart inflammation from Covid).

Phillips was on a high-flow nasal cannula that morning; he could talk and even eat a little. His main comment was that he was really hungry, giving me a crooked smile. When I asked if he was having any trouble breathing, he said: "No doc – my oxygen level falls when I take this thing off (indicating the nasal cannula), but I feel good. Just keep wondering when my lunch is coming."

"It's on its way Phillips, but I'm not sure exactly when." The wall clock indicated it was 12:15. *His lunch was late.* We gabbed a little, and Phillips offered the story of how he got to our hospital.

"I live with my Mom and Dad – take care of them. We all got Covid the same time, but my dad got it the worst. We tried to just wait it out at home, and hunker down, but it got to where my dad couldn't even get out of bed anymore. So I decided to bring him to the hospital. He was too sick to walk, so I had to carry him out to our car like he was a little kid." He held his forearms out, palms facing up, to show how he did it. "There was this much snow on the ground" – now holding his hands about a foot apart. "Took me 90 minutes to drive to Winslow in our pickup. But I was having a lot of trouble myself, breathing, I mean. Almost felt like I was underwater. And I remembered when I was a kid, my parents made me take swimming lessons. They taught me how to breathe when I was swimming, and I concentrated on that, to keep breathing while I was driving." He held his hands, palms facing his chest and took some deep breaths to show me. "I just concentrated on my breathing and we made it to the ER in Winslow. So anyway, that's my story Doc. Now hey, can you please check on how that lunch is coming?"

Prayer 208 (February 10, 2021)
Father, you said: "I took you from the ends of the Earth, from its farthest corners I called you.
I said you are my children I have chosen you.
So do not fear, for I am with you.
I will strengthen and help you in your time of need.
I will uphold you with my righteous right hand."
[From Isaiah 41:9-10.]

Jesus, you said do not worry – all our worries cannot add a single hour to our life.
Help us not be discouraged.
Help us trust you 100%.
Give Phillips, Daisy and Lee your peace today.
Day by day you are carrying us down a rocky road, but it is your road. You are in charge.
You invite us to pray to you so we can share in your miracles.
You brought us together to witness your healing power.
The day is coming soon when we will be safe again by your

command, and we will give thanks and praise in your holy name!

Daisy happily responded by text today that Lee was doing OK with his new trach, was awake, responding to simple commands and nodding yes/no appropriately to her and the nurses!

Back at work, I picked up the care of a Covid patient named Sabrina, who had been on *piperacillin/tazobactam* and vancomycin* antibiotics for the last nine days. Looking back through the chart, I could see why they were started – she had spiked a fever of 101.8° on her sixth ICU day. In such cases, we cultured blood and ETT secretions and started antibiotics until the culture results were known. In this case, the cultures were all negative. Other lab values showed no evidence of ongoing bacterial infection, and even if there had been, nine days of antibiotics should have treated it. A clear case for antibiotic stewardship; I discontinued the antibiotics.

Two days later, Sabrina spiked a fever to 103° and developed worsening oxygenation. Joyce re-cultured her and restarted the same antibiotics I had just discontinued.

[*Tazobactam, like the aforementioned avibactam, is not an antibiotic per se, but a synthetic enzyme that digests the antibiotic-resistance enzymes produced by some bacteria – essentially an escalation of the chemical warfare waged between the bacteria and our drug development scientists!]*

Prayer 209 (February 12, 2021)
We did not ask for this room or this music. We were invited here.
We have been surrounded by darkness so that we would turn our faces to the light.
We have endured hardship to learn to be grateful for blessings.
We have been threatened by defeat to be astounded by miracles.
We have been born in sin to be amazed by God's mercy.
We have been given life to defy death.
We did not ask for this room or this music, but since God invited us

together here, let us dance for him.
[This was a quote from Steven King that I took the liberty of repurposing as a prayer]

Sabrina developed septic shock. Her blood and ETT secretion cultures grew *S. aureus* sensitive to vancomycin – the same antibiotic she had been on for nine days, that I discontinued only 48 hours before she crashed. I looked back through the chart, and even presented the case to a infectious disease consultant, thinking perhaps I had made a mistake discontinuing antibiotics. Neither of us could find any error with that decision except that it turned out to be wrong. That didn't keep it from weighing heavily on my conscience during the weeks after Sabrina passed, and still sometimes until this very day.

Prayer 210 (February 18, 2021)
If God is with us, who can be against us?
He who did not even spare his own Son, but gave him up for us – will he not also graciously give us all good things?
Christ Jesus is the one who died and who was raised – who is at the right hand of God interceding for us!
Who shall separate us from the love of Christ?
[Reprise Romans 8:31-35]

After Lee regained the ability to talk again in late March, he told me the worst thing that ever happened to him, happened around this date. As was often the case, Lee found himself wide awake at 3 am – his circadian rhythm completely discombobulated by his residence in the ICU – when his nurse left the room for a moment. Just as she stepped out, the tubing connecting his tracheostomy to the ventilator popped off and fell to the floor. He couldn't reach it, couldn't cry out for help because of the tracheostomy, couldn't find the call button, lost in the bedsheets somewhere. He couldn't breathe. HE PANICKED. As he desperately groped for the lost call button, he could feel himself greying-out from lack of oxygen. "I thought that was the end of me!"

Just then, the nurse stepped back into the room in time to rush over and put him back on the vent*. The memory of this near-death experience subsequently recurred every time Lee's nurse left the room, psychologically haunting him in the months ahead. It's understandable that as many as a third of ICU patients subsequently develop post-traumatic stress disorder – an injury even an experienced doctor like Lee cannot rationally minimize. [*I later learned that Lee had experienced a fullblown cardiopulmonary arrest during this episode.*]

Prayer 211 (February 19, 2021)
"In the beginning was the word, and the word was with God, and the word was God."
Thank you for your word Lord Jesus.
When you speak, miracles happen.
When we listen to your word, we find peace, wisdom and forgiveness.
Open our ears tonight Lord, as we lay in bed; let us hear your word and be blessed by it.

Our Covid census slowly began to diminish again, mainly due to accumulating fatality. During one of my infrequent night shifts, I admitted a 98-year-woman with heart failure who remarkably did *not* have Covid. She was white-haired and a little forgetful but not nearly as frail as I imagined when I first heard received report from the ER. Upon meeting her, I noticed a crude numeric tattoo on her left forearm: "26068."

It was 1 am, and she wasn't here to tell me stories about the Holocaust. I should at least take care of her medically before asking her about that concentration camp tattoo. But when I was done with my history and physical, she seemed in no distress and not adverse to talking a little more. So I asked her. "Sarah, can you tell me <u>one</u> thing about this? – lightly touching the tattoo.

"Vat do you want me to tell you?" (she spoke loudly, as though I might be hard-of-hearing).

I didn't know what to ask; I figured it was best to let her decide.

"You survived such a horrible experience; teach me one important thing that I can learn from you."

She was silent for a moment. "Well . . . it was a *miracle.* That's one thing. There were seven of us. My mother was 46 years of age. I was seventeen. My youngest brother was three. And I was the only one who survived the camps. I don't know how. I don't know why. I don't remember *what I did* to survive. I just did. It was a miracle."

"A miracle? A miracle sounds like something that God does. Do you believe in God, Sarah?" She gave me an enigmatic, knowing smile and no further answer. I subsequently pondered the significance of her expression many times without a firm conclusion.

Sarah recovered from heart failure quickly and was discharged two days later.

I worked out that Sarah was 17 years old in 1940 when the women's concentration camp at Auschwitz-Birkenau opened. Tattooing of women prisoners of Auschwitz-Birkenau began later, in 1942. At first, concentration camp prisoners were given clothing that had identification numbers sewn onto them. The camps switched to tattoos because they had trouble keeping track of the identity of dead bodies after they were stripped naked. Her tattoo number, 26068, indicated that 26,067 women had received concentration camp tattoos before Sarah. One million, one-hundred-thousand people – mostly Jewish – were murdered at Auschwitz. *Amazingly, some deny it ever happened.*

It somehow wasn't surprising that Sarah was unaffected by Covid after all she had been through in life. A great privilege of working in medicine is the opportunity to meet wondrous survivors who have fought their way through history, like Sarah.

Prayer 212 (February 20, 2021)
Glory and praise to you, O God, Creator and Sustainer of life,

Inventor of light and love.
Merciful Father and humble Son, who suffered and died to make a
clear pathway to Heaven for us, Great Healer. Consoler of those in
sorrow, Giver of Peace to those burdened by worry, preserve us!

Lee had now survived five weeks in the ICU. By this time, most Covid pneumonia patients would have either recovered or died, but Lee was stuck in limbo. He required 80% oxygen. A CT lung scan showed extensive destruction of the delicate architecture of the lungs, now largely replaced with scar tissue, making his lungs stiff – incredibly hard to inflate. The ventilator pressure required to allow Lee even a shallow breath was consequently dangerously high. Research had shown that it was distinctly unusual for active Covid infection to persist beyond three weeks, but the damage already done to Lee's lungs was so severe that he was having trouble naturally recovering from it. To make matters worse, severe anxiety was wearing him out, and he had to be re-sedated

A lung CT showing
severe lung scarring
(white areas) due to
Covid pneumonia.

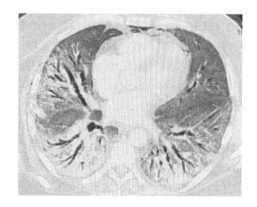

Prayer 213 (February 22, 2021)
I was thinking of this yesterday; I don't know if it counts as a prayer or not: but there is no such thing as a setback to you God.
You cannot be surprised or disappointed in anything that happens.

Nothing can stand in the way of your will.
You never take your eye off the ball.
Lord, if you say "Lee, get up out of that hospital bed and go home,"
that is what will happen – in your timing.
We will not be shaken because our protector is the Lord!

Our census finally fell to 26 today after having spent 94 days above our "maximum safe census." Only eight of our remaining ICU patients had Covid.

Prayer 214 (February 27, 2021)
Jesus – fan into flame our God-given faith, for you gave us a spirit of power and love, not fear!
Therefore we are not ashamed of the testimony of our Lord, because you called us to a holy vocation by your grace.
And you created us to serve your purpose, which you planned before the beginning of time. [Paraphrase of 2 Timothy 1:6-9].

We are not afraid or ashamed to beg you Lord, on our knees, to heal all still suffering from Covid.
We don't care what others think of us, we only have our eyes on you.
Your will be done.
We thank you for every moment of life you give us.

When I returned to work after five days off, the ICU seemed palpably different. I looked down my new patient list; many of the names were now unfamiliar. The names of my previous patients were quickly fading from memory, *perhaps as a defense mechanism*. I walked briskly around the unit to get a feel for the service and say hi to a few of the nurses. One of the pods had been closed and many of the remaining patients were shuffled into new rooms. Empty proning beds, cleaned and plastic-wrapped, lined the hallways. As I walked by a room, I saw a patient I didn't recognize with a white beard and short dark black hair. I could see from the ventilator control panel in the hall that he was doing poorly on 100% oxygen and very high ventilator pressures.

About an hour later, as I was working my way down the list of patients I had been assigned, I realized that the man I didn't recognize earlier was Phillips! He'd grown a beard since last I saw him and had badly deteriorated. It seemed purposefully spiteful – one last stab at our hearts as Covid waned.

There were no proven Covid therapies Phillips hadn't already received. But I started him on high-dose dexamethasone same as I did for Hurley. I started three antimicrobials in an attempt to prevent secondary infections that might exploit the immunosuppression caused by such high-dose dexamethasone – *antibiotic stewardship be darned.* Isaiah came into the room and joined me as I prayed aloud at Phillip's bedside.

Prayer 215 (February 28, 2021)
Lord Jesus – the Great Healer.
God the Father – you have providence over everything in Heaven and on Earth, yet you have heard our prayer, and you smiled on us. Keep your miracle coming Lord.
We are not asking for anything less than all we desire for Phillips and for Lee because we know your word is law.
Just say the word again today merciful Father.
Heal them! Get them home to their family and friends.
We give you thanks and praise. We will never forget this miracle.

Lee had been started on a protocol to wean him off the ventilator by gradually reducing his ventilator pressures over weeks, allowing him to take back over the work of breathing little by little. This usually succeeded as a patient's lungs healed. But if Lee's lungs *weren't* healing, the protocol assured that he would have to work just a little bit harder for each breath he took with each passing day.

After work today, I went for a run, took a shower and shared a nice dinner with Jean: homemade pizza topped with sauteed artichoke hearts and Italian sausage – a glass of Chianti. But I couldn't help thinking of Philips and Lee, in the ICU, on ventilators, tube feedings being pumped into their stomachs through a nasogastric tube. Every moment of a normal day is an incredible blessing that should not be taken for granted. I bet those guys would give *anything* right now just to be sitting on their couch at home eating dinner and watching TV with their families as I was.

Lord, we thank you for life – for all the myriad blessings that go into each day here at home on Earth.
If it wasn't for serious illness, we would never realize how precious they are.
Lord, please open our eyes so we can see your love influencing every moment of our lives!

Prayer 216 (March 1, 2021)
Jesus, firstborn brother, help me pick up my cross and follow you.
Because those the Father foreknew, he also predestined to be conformed to your image.
And since you predestined this for me, you justified me and you will glorify me forever – none of which I could ever deserve, except that all things obey your will and grace.
And what then can I say in response?
"If God is for me, who can be against me!"
Thank you for making me who I am.
[Based on Romans 8:29-31]

I think few people who work outside the hospital fully appreciate how enduring and forgiving ICU nurses can be. They are very special people. I think of (most of) them as the closest things to everyday angels living on Earth – *with the possible inclusion of grammar-school teachers.*

Today we admitted a lady who weighed 475 lbs. for respiratory failure due to obesity. It was physically very difficult for her to use a bedpan, so she told the nurses she wouldn't use one. The nurses had to clean her and change her bedsheets each time she had a bowel movement. They did this with compassion and without recrimination.

Some years ago, one of our nurses got married sporting a black eye given to her a few days earlier by an alcoholic patient with delirium tremens. Her explanation: "Well, I know he didn't *mean it* – he wasn't himself that day; he was sick."

Our nurses never once refrained from joining prayer in a patient's room when invited to do so. Although I'm sure many are not Christian, they seem to always be willing to put the patient's needs before their own.

Prayer 217 (March 2, 2021)
Praise our heavenly Father, from whom all good things come.
Please bless the nurses Lord Jesus.
They follow so closely in your footsteps.
They come to serve, just as you did.
They are not too proud to do any tough or dirty task.
They don't complain.
They are fair but compassionate and forgiving.
Lord, please bless all nurses.
Give them strength to go on, and encourage them that their hard work makes a difference, in this world and the next.

Prayer 218 (March 3, 2021)
What may be known about you God, you have made plain, because you have made your presence in our world obvious.
For since the creation of the world, your eternal power and divine nature have been clearly seen.
We thank you, Lord for being conspicuously present in the lives of those you have graciously chosen so that our faith can be strengthened in all circumstances.
We thank you for loving Lee and Daisy and blessing them.
Covid is too strong for us, but it's nothing compared to your sovereign power.
Say the word Lord!
[Derived from Romans 1]

Our census was down to 23 patients - and only three with Covid.

Maryam was the last of our Covid patients to die during the winter surge. A 65-year-old Algerian woman, she and many other members of her family caught Covid from each other attending her daughter Basma's wedding ceremony in Egypt. In the hospital, her devout Muslim family worked as a tag team to provide Maryam with constant bedside attendance – there was no way in or out of the ICU without bumping into one of them and being asked how Maryam was doing. Unfortunately, the news went from bad to worse. Zahra (Maryam's sister), dressed in a plain aba and hijab, was the family spokesperson, "We are like the same person – my sister Maryam and I. I know what she is thinking. If you want to know how she is feeling, doctor, ask me – I'll tell you." But communication with her family was hindered by language, religious and cultural differences; they believed that assent to DNR status or comfort care was inconsistent with their Muslim faith.

Maryam's right lung ruptured and cultures from her ETT grew *Pseudomonas aeruginosa* bacteria. In the ensuing 48 hours, her O2 sats inexorably fell until, on the last day of her life, they reached 20% – *seemingly incompatible with even momentary life.* Somehow her heart kept beating as her husband Sami and sister Zahra sat at her bedside holding her hands, having mercifully been granted an exception to our visitation restrictions through the kindness of our administrators and nurses. I felt permission to ask them to pray together. I was just a little worried about how they might feel praying with a Christian, but they accepted without hesitation.

Father God – we are all your children.
We come together now under your shadow to pray for Maryam.
She is your daughter the one whom you love.
And she loves you Father –
Do not let her be put to shame for her faith in you.
Hear our prayer Lord.
Heal her. Protect her.

Surround her in your mighty arms and she will not be afraid. Hold her Lord, and bless her according to her faith in you, which is great.

Father, hear the tears of her family.

Bless her daughter Basma.
Bless Sami and Zahra.
Give them strength and keep them by your side.
Do a miracle for them, for your glory.
We give you all thanks, all praise.
We know all good things only come from you.
In your holy name we pray.

Is it OK for a Christian to pray to the Father with people from other faiths who don't believe in Jesus?

I don't know. But I listen to my gut when I consider praying with a patient or their family, and I trust the Holy Spirit to guide me. And I've always felt an affinity to people of faith regardless of their religion. *Sojourners with the same destination share a certain kinship, even if they travel different paths.* There is no way to the Father except through the Son, but judgment is God's alone, and Jesus can make pathways of salvation far beyond my human comprehension. And Jesus once said, "For whoever is not against us is for us." [Mark 9:40] Only God can judge who is for him, and who against. If it makes any sense to pray *for a prayer*, that's what I did – *Jesus, let this prayer be acceptable in your eyes.*

I included Maryam's daughter Basma in our prayer with the hope she might be unburdened by any guilt over the circumstances under which Maryam fell ill. Covid robbed us of family traditions, religious ceremonies and cultural rites or tainted them with death. Maryam caught Covid on her daughter's wedding day – supposed to have been one of the happiest days of their life. Now, the memory would always carry a horrible footnote – her family deprived even of the weak consolation of a proper funeral for Maryam.

Prayer 219 (March 7, 2021)

I thank you Lord, that the harder something is for us, the closer you get.

As you heal our brothers and sisters, I pray that the incredible faith that you have invested in them, in their hour of gravest peril, will not fade as they recover and return home.

And we also pray for those who are blind to your authority and loving-kindness.

Let their suffering lead them to your feet, and bless them not only with medical healing but with the healing of their spirits, bringing them into your loving arms.

Lee texted me the simple message: "On vent." It was the first text I received from him in two months. At first I thought it was a weird text – *maybe he was delirious* – but then I realized, like most ICU patients, Lee probably had little memory of what had happened to him. Noting that he was "On vent" was perhaps the most astute medical observation he could have made. Being on the vent for two months was distinctly unusual and foreboding. Maybe he was beginning to wonder whether he would ever come off. Daisy told me later that two physical therapists stood Lee up that afternoon and even helped him take a few steps using especially long ventilator tubing. His mental status was definitely recovering.

Prayer 220 (March 13, 2021)

Thanks Lord for sending us all the things we need for life each day –fresh air, sunshine, rain and snow to water the Earth, trees to make oxygen, wind to make the trees move, animals to live under their branches . . .all the natural world you made to nurture us, and surround us with beauty, and remind us that you, the Great Creator, love us and are present all around us always.

March 16, 2021. *An ancient-appearing alligator juniper frosted with snow shortly after sunrise, Payson, AZ.*

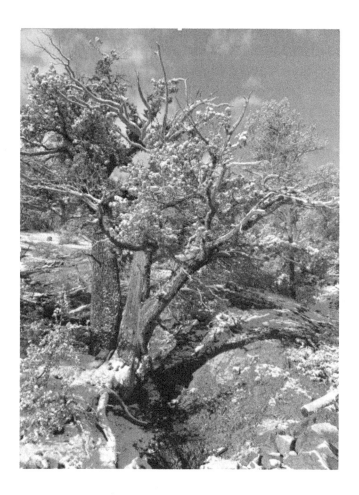

Prayer 221 (March 15, 2021)

I worked the last couple of nights and my mind was still too fuzzy to think of a good prayer. But I remembered last night at about 2 am, I had just finished seeing a new patient and was worn out. I lay down in the call room bed and tried to relax, but I could hear all kinds of action going on through the call room door: alarms going off, people coughing, people gabbing like it was 2 in the afternoon – I simply prayed by calling out to the Father:

"Hear me Father.
Do not forsake me.
I am here."

The next thing I knew, it was 6 am. Four hours without a page! I thank God for giving us pleasure in the provision of what our bodies need.

As Lee progressed through the ventilator weaning protocol, he took on more and more of the work of breathing but just couldn't ever seem to make it all the way off the vent. Although he was receiving almost 4000 calories of tube feeds per day (a normal diet for a man his size is about 2000–2400 calories), he was progressively losing weight. Metabolic analysis showed that Lee was burning 5000 calories a day! From what I understand, marathon runners utilize about 100 cal/mile or about 2600 cal/marathon. That meant that Lee's work of breathing was the caloric equivalent of running a marathon every day! Lee was a fighter, but no human being could endure this level of continuous stress. Lee's physicians decided to give up on Lee ever being weaned off the ventilator. It had now been two months. His lungs were clearly never going to recover. They ramped ventilator support back up so that he could nutritionally recover while they considered plan B.

Prayer 222 (March 17, 2021)
Whatever is good upon this Earth
is only a shadow of greatness in Heaven.
What a great sense of humor you two must have, Father and Son.
Thanks for the little spark of it you put in us, who have been made in your image.
Thanks for reminding us occasionally of the carefree days of childhood (for those of us blessed with such memories), when getting an Oscar Meyer whistle was one of life's exciting little pleasures.

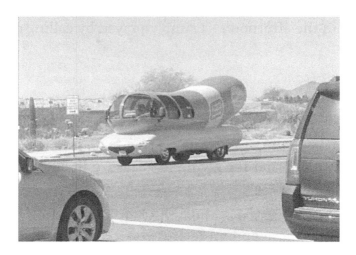

We passed the Oscar Meyer Weinermobile on the road today (Jean was driving, so I was able to take a photo safely). Jean started singing that old advertizing ditty: "Oh, I wish I were an Oscar Mayer Weiner – that is what I truly want to be. 'Cuz if I was an Oscar Mayer Weiner, everyone would be in love with me!"

A wife with a good sense of humor is a great blessing! Remember what it was like to be a kid? – how excited could you get over a silly little thing like getting an Oscar Meyer hotdog whistle? I loved that I could still see the little kid in Jean.

Prayer 223 (March 18, 2021)
Heavenly Father hear our praise.
The life you gave us was not meant to be easy, but rather to glorify you.
We have all been through our own version of hard times.
When we are in the midst of suffering, we are anxious about what our future holds.
But when we look back, it's clear that you were always there for us; you never abandoned us.
No matter what, you always heard our prayers.
This time is no different.
Bless us Lord. Say we will all be healed.

Let your name once again be glorified.
Bolster our courage and faith in the hard times ahead, and let your
will for us be done, no matter the earthly situation.

I had let several technicalities lapse during the first year of Covid. One of these was the completion of mandatory educational modules required to maintain my clinical status at the hospital where I previously worked. This status was important to my research, so I had to backtrack and get my computer access reinstated and complete the modules. A very nice person named Dawn helped me get a new username and password to start the process, which I fancifully thought would allow me to easily complete the modules remotely from home.

I opened the site, entered the username and password and got an "incorrect username/password" message. I re-entered it, making sure I spelled everything correctly, with the proper capitalization. Incorrect. I looked back at the instructions – they indicated that you had to enter a domain with your username, giving examples of adding the domain name both as a prefix *and* as a suffix. So I tried it one way, then the other: incorrect and incorrect.

I checked that I had used the backslash/forward slash correctly and tried again. Incorrect. I called the help desk and navigated through many levels of the automated phone menu, eventually reaching a recording that told me the wait time for help was 51 minutes. I waited for about 20 minutes, during which time I tried many other sign-on permutations, eventually prompting a message that my account was now locked.

I decided it would ultimately be more effective to simply drive into the hospital; in-house computers sometimes worked better for this sort of thing due to security firewalls. But when I arrived around noon, I couldn't get into the parking lot because my ID card had expired. I parked out in a remote lot and walked over to the security office to get an updated ID badge, but it was locked-up, and there was a sign on the door that they were (already) closed for the day – *it was only 10:45 am!* – There was a smiley face on the sign.

I walked over to an office I used to share in an older section of the hospital. The door still had an old-fashioned lock, and my key still worked! I got behind a hospital computer and tried the username and password in several iterations again with no success. I called the help desk and a recorded message came informing me the wait time was now *58 minutes!* My phone pinged and displayed the beginning of a text: Inez: "Hello, Sorry to bother you." I was getting pretty frustrated by this time. I had one simple job to do: <u>finish my mandatory educational modules</u>, and I needed to stay focused if I was ever going to get it done!

But the text was from my old friend and patient Inez.

Seeing her name on my phone display helped me take a deep breath and refocus: *remember who the real Boss is.*

Inez texted again: "Are you at the hospital right now?" *She meant the hospital I used to work at when I took care of her so many years ago, the same hospital I happened to be sitting inside at the moment.* I hadn't worked here in four years, but I just happened to be on campus when I received her text.

Inez: "One of our firefighters with Covid will be taken off life support there this afternoon."

I called her. A fellow firefighter named Santiago was in the ICU with terminal Covid pneumonia. I shared the remarkable "coincidence" by which I happened to be at the hospital and asked her what she wanted me to do.

"I don't know what you *can* do. I just heard about what was happening with Santiago and got this feeling that I should call you." She paused, "Could you go pray with the family? I remember how we prayed together all those years ago and how much it helped me and my mother. I think it would mean the world to Santiago's family. His wife Elena is at his bedside now, and I can let her know you're coming."

OK. Now I know why I'm sitting here at this computer terminal.

"Sure, Inez, I'll go up there and see what I can do. I'll call you later – say hi to Nate."

I called the operator and got Santiago's room number. I went to the security desk in the ER and told the guard that I was a doctor trying to see a patient in the ICU, but my ID card was expired. (I should note that I was wearing jeans and a T-shirt and hadn't shaved in several days, not having expected to go visit a patient. I wasn't sure whether he would believe my story.)

Security said, "No problem doc, I'll take you right up." When we entered the locked unit together using his security ID, two nurses, neither of whom I had seen in four years, immediately recognized me despite my face mask and warmly greeted me, validating my identity for the security guard. Santiago's nurse was another surprised old friend, and when I told her I was there to pray, she replied, "Good, this family really needs it."

I looked into Santiago's room. He had an ECMO tubing half as large as a garden hose sutured into the jugular vein of his neck, feeding oxygen-rich blood directly into his lungs and heart. He was deeply sedated, surrounded by a spider web of IV lines and monitor cables. But I could easily imagine him standing up straight and tall in his firefighter gear. On the other side of the bed, gowned and masked, were two women, one with her arm over the other's shoulder. By coincidence, both were named Elena, Santiago's wife and a fellow firefighter from his crew. I felt no awkwardness explaining the situation to them – why I was there, a complete stranger, a doctor from another hospital, come to the ICU bedside specifically to pray with them. I had no doubt that they would agree to pray, as it appeared quite clear to me that God's work was afoot and would not be turned aside by any act of man or computer. With Santiago's wife Elena's permission, I gowned and gloved up and went to the right bedside across from the two Elenas. We all laid hands on Santiago together and prayed.

Prayer 224 (March 20, 2021)

O Lord, be my shepherd.
Free me from want and worry.
Lead me back to your garden, let me find rest there in the meadow,
and peace beside its tranquil waters.
Heal my errant soul.
Make me righteous in your sight through the blood of your Son, for
the glory of the Father.
When I find myself surrounded by evil, when it seems my very life is
imperiled, fill me with courage, because you, the almighty, are my
protector!
In dire calamity, do not forsake me, but acknowledge me before all,
as you would your son, and pour down your blessing on me.
Grant me your loving-kindness and mercy, and gather me into your
holy presence for all eternity.

March 2021. Hiking the Peralta trail with Carlos.

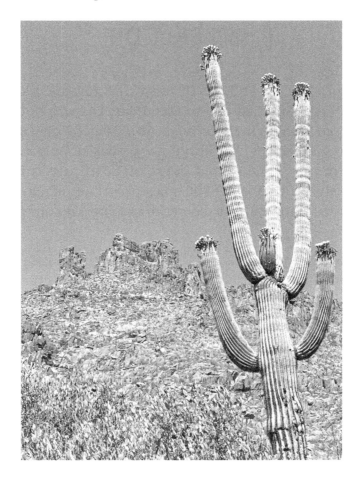

INTERLUDE

By April 2021, over 3,600 US nurses, doctors and healthcare support staff had died due to Covid, but Lee was not among them. And although there were 68 distinct Covid hospital outbreaks in Arizona, our hospital was spared. Only a handful of our nurses caught mild cases of Covid. God's blessing was surely on that old P100 mask of mine, which (I have forewarned Jean) will one day retire to hang over our fireplace mantel.

Up to this point, our ICU team had taken care of 663 Covid pneumonia patients, who cumulatively accrued 4,621 ICU days over a single year. They ranged from 18 to 92 years old. Some had many severe comorbid risk factors, and some were previously healthy. Our primary immunosuppressive treatments, such as dexamethasone – *proven effective in well-conducted clinical trials* – seemed to have little discernable benefit once a patient started down the terminal path of severe respiratory failure and all its complications: ruptured lungs, kidney failure and secondary bacterial pneumonia. Three hundred fifteen of our patients died from Covid, 206 during the summer and winter Covid surges alone. This makes an average of over one Covid death per day in our ICU, every day for six months.

Covid ICU survivors were reduced to a shell of their former selves. We lost track of many but were aware that some endured the unit only to die shortly thereafter in nursing homes and rehab centers. But Phillips, the young Native American man who used his childhood swimming lessons to help himself breathe while driving his father to an emergency room, was an exception. Phillips slowly recovered and eventually returned home to take care of his mother.

God performed another spectacular miracle healing Lee, the sickest Covid patient I have ever known to survive. Although the damage Covid inflicted on his lungs was apparently irreparable, Lee stubbornly refused to give up and slowly gained back some weight. In late April, on the 94th day of his illness, he was deemed fit enough to receive a double lung transplant.

Prayer 225 (April 28, 2021)
Father, who created our bodies molecule by molecule, smile on the efforts of your children to emulate you – the Great Healer.
Bless this pair of lungs Lee has received Lord!
Breathe into them and fill them with life.
Our trust is 100% only in you.
Lord Jesus, you are worthy of our trust – so worthy.
You are the Hearer of Prayers.
The Consoler of the Suffering.
The one whose slightest touch heals all disease.
We love you Lord. We thank you.
You do not disappoint the faithful.
All praise to you for getting Lee through this valley
of the shadow of death. All thanks and glory to you!

A week after his lung transplant, Lee was up walking again, pushing his ventilator down the hall. Two weeks later, he ate real food again for the first time in four months (if you call green Jell-O "food"). On May 30th, Lee and Daisy celebrated their 40th wedding anniversary in the healing garden of the hospital. His tracheostomy was removed and he breathed free air for the first time in four and a half months! On June 10th, Lee went home after 143 days in the hospital. A hundred healthcare workers lined the hallway out to the hospital parking lot, cheering him and his family on as they left the hospital and headed home. Thank God for blessing us with this great miracle; let it be for his glory! We prayed and you answered. What a great way to end this book. I sincerely thought the story was over, but I was wrong once again.

June 10, 2021. *Lee sitting in his walker with his grandson in his lap, waiting for Daisy to bring the car around and take him home from the hospital after a 143-day admission.*

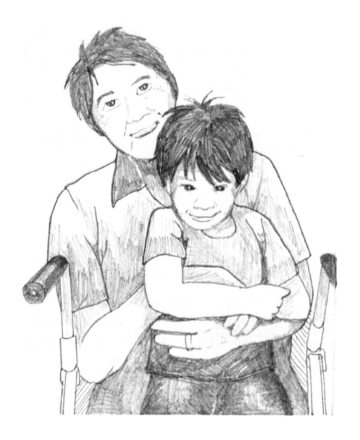

DELTA AND OMICRON SURGE 2021-22: FORGIVENESS

Covid receded during the spring and early summer of 2021 as community vaccination progressed. By mid-July 2021, our ICU was again briefly free of Covid pneumonia – *this time, I thought, for good.* We saw occasional readmissions: long Covid patients with crippled lungs and severe physical debilitation presenting with complications of prolonged residence in healthcare facilities including pressure sores, urinary catheter infections, infectious diarrhea . . .

But in early August, a harbinger of ill tidings arrived – an acute manifestation of Covid we had never seen before. A 23-year-old woman was admitted with moderate Covid pneumonia requiring oxygen. Within an hour of admission, she experienced a grand mal seizure and a "stroke alert" was called, triggering an emergent brain CT to look for bleeding or blockage of a cerebral blood vessel, *unlikely as either might be in a 23-year-old.* The CT scan was normal. She was sleepy thereafter, as is typical after a grand mal seizure, and lay quietly in bed the rest of the day. But around midnight, she lapsed into a coma and began experiencing aspiration: saliva running down her windpipe into her lungs without triggering any neurological impulse to cough. She was intubated and aggressively suctioned to clear her airways. A repeat CT showed severe brain swelling. A twin-lobed structure deep in the brain called the thalamus – *the central relay centers and the seat of consciousness* – had catastrophically hemorrhaged. There was little we could do as she inexorably progressed to brain death by 6 am the following morning – only 20 hours after being admitted! Fatal Covid brain involvement was rare, but well-documented in the literature. Our brilliant neurologist, Dr. Richards (who had once cheered us with his wild ride through the ICU on the floor-cleaning Zamboni), suggested that this case might be due to the Delta Covid variant.

The Delta variant, first identified in India, was 50% more contagious than the previous Alpha variant of Covid, rapidly supplanting it. Covid cases began rising by late July and were surging by August. By mid-Sept, the daily Covid case rate in Arizona rivaled that during the catastrophic summer surge of 2020.

Vaccination had not gone as well as expected. Over 600,000 Americans had died from Covid and the vaccine had been shown to reduce mortality by 95%. Yet by September 2021, nine months after Covid vaccine became available, less than half of Arizonans were fully vaccinated. Many people were more afraid of the vaccine than they were of Covid.

This made absolutely no sense from our perspective in the ICU. Consider that practically every person with a life-threatening medical disease or complication ends up in the ICU and that <u>we had seen hundreds of patients with fatal Covid pneumonia but not a single patient with critically illness due to a vaccine complication.</u>

Even *before* Covid, the majority of adult ICU admissions were at least partially self-inflicted, due to alcoholism, drug use, morbid obesity, and smoking. I've often felt that our specialty would scarcely exist if people led healthy lifestyles. Everyone who works in the ICU has learned to accept this. But after experiencing 18 months of suffering and death alongside hundreds of patients and their families, the renewed influx of unvaccinated Covid pneumonia patients was almost more than we could bear. These stubbornly misinformed people invited disaster upon themselves and were taking us down with them.

The Delta surge was largely comprised of a new type of Covid patient: politically-conservative Christians like me! One of our nurses, a horse owner raised in rural Arizona, described them with exasperation as "our tribe." Vaccination had unfortunately become a political issue, conservatives standing against. A member of the Texas House of Representatives, who supported Covid mask-burning events and called a physician promoting vaccination "an enemy of free people,"

was admitted for Covid pneumonia on August 1st and died on a ventilator three days later, leaving behind a widow and baby son. Delta Covid pneumonia patients entering our ICU were practically all strident anti-vaxxers who distrusted the establishment (represented by my partners and me) and believed we were purposely withholding effective Covid treatments promoted on social media. From August 2021 through the end of this story in February 2022, 95% of all the Covid patients we took care of in the ICU had purposefully chosen to remain unvaccinated – *a choice which increased the mortality risk from Covid thirty times!* Our ICU team had a new internal struggle to deal with: overcoming our anger.

Prayer 226 (August 10, 2021)
Thank you Father, that your word is alive and active.
Sharper than any sword, it penetrates even to dividing soul and spirit, joints and marrow.
By your word are the thoughts and attitudes of my heart measured.
Nothing in all creation is hidden from you.
Everything is uncovered and laid bare before your eyes.
How can I stand?
Praise Jesus, the Son of God, the Highest Priest, ascended into Heaven.
Help me hold fast your gift of faith.
Jesus, you empathize with us in our human weakness, having been tempted in every way, yet you did not sin!
Thanks to you, Lord Jesus, who I even dare call my "Brother."
I can approach God's throne with confidence only because of your sacrifice, and receive your mercy and grace in my time of need.

[From Hebrews 4:12-14]

We had a memorable non-Covid case before the Delta surge went into full swing: a 25-year-old man named Hector who overdosed on fentanyl in a parking garage. The high in Phoenix was 110 degrees that day and Hector was found in a coma, barely breathing, with a body temperature of 107 degrees – a condition called "heat stroke." EMS administered Narcan (the antidote to fentanyl and other narcotics) with no effect. Hector was intubated and rapidly cooled in our ER. His wife and Spanish-speaking mother arrived in the ICU shortly thereafter; both remarkably intelligent and loving. If you had only met *them*, you would never suspect that Hector's predicament was self-inflicted. They related Hector had overdosed before, but there was no recrimination in their attitude. They were both simply focused on seeing him recover.

But over the first three days of his admission, Hector remained comatose – only minimally reactive to pain. He was stuck on a ventilator until he awoke – *if he awoke*. Whenever I encounter heat stroke related to drug abuse, I remember the old TV commercial – "This is your brain. This is your brain on drugs." Heat stroke denatures proteins in the brain and I couldn't help but worry Hector might have "fried his egg."

Later that day, I noticed Hector's family had covered him with a pink faux-fur children's blanket with a rainbow-colored unicorn printed on it. The family told me this belonged to Hector's two-year-old daughter Anabelle. I asked them to bring in a picture of Anabelle to hang on the wall, so that Hector could see it when he awoke – *and to encourage the empathy of Hector's doctors and nurses, including myself.*

Prayer 227 (August 13, 2021)
I have to stop for a moment and ask you Lord to soften my hard heart.
The craziness in the world around me is killing my compassion.
This morning Lord, make in me a new heart.

Shelter me from Satan's attacks.
Let your Holy Spirit burn bright in me Lord.
Let me never see a patient as anything less than a brother or sister in pain*, and let me be a blessing to them, no matter how they got here.
Hear my cry my Father and rescue me!

I held a Zoom meeting that week to discuss compassion fatigue with some medical students. One of the students related something her supervising resident taught her about the care of patients with substance abuse disorders in the ICU: "Don't try any harder than the patient." *Essentially, if the patient doesn't care about themselves, neither should you.*

But I told the students that it's our job in the ICU to try and give people another chance at life without fretting over what they might do with it. We all need second chances. This requires giving the patient the benefit of the doubt and always doing our job to the best of our ability. I also reminded them to consider the patients' family and friends, who suffer alongside and count on us.

[*This phrase comes from the Oath of Maimonides, a prayer written by a twelfth-century Jewish physician that best articulates the attitude that a physician should aspire to obtain. Unfortunately, few medical schools have students recite this oath anymore, but I have had the opportunity to share it with incoming medical students every year when I speak to them about the vocation of medicine. And I love to personally review it during challenging times. It seems proof of divine influence when a statement of purpose like this transcends the ages with enduring relevance.]*

The Oath of Maimonides:
"The eternal providence has appointed me to watch over the life and health of Thy creatures.
May the love for my art actuate me at all times; may neither avarice nor miserliness nor thirst for glory or for a great reputation

engage my mind; for the enemies of truth and philanthropy could easily deceive me and make me forgetful of my lofty aim of doing good to Thy children.

May I never see in the patient anything but a fellow creature in pain.

Grant me the strength, time and opportunity always to correct what I have acquired, always to extend its domain; for knowledge is immense and the spirit of man can extend indefinitely to enrich itself daily with new requirements.

Today he can discover his errors of yesterday and tomorrow he can obtain a new light on what he thinks himself sure of today.

Oh, God, Thou has appointed me to watch over the life and death of Thy creatures; here am I ready for my vocation and now I turn unto my calling."

Prayer 228 (August 18, 2021)
Jesus, when you were here on Earth as a human, you loved people.
You loved little children and they loved you.
You upheld the humble.
You were homeless but wouldn't send a friend home hungry.
You hung out with the rejects.
You never used your power to help yourself, only others.
You healed everyone who asked.
You didn't seek the approval of men but of God.
You were completely honest and forthright, even when it had fatal personal consequences.
You did not abide religious hypocrisy.
You never lost your temper from insult or injury, but only when the Father was disrespected.
You didn't seek social status, political authority or technology to amplify your voice, but you spoke straight to the hearts of individuals you personally touched.
You were scared about what God asked you to do, but you did it anyway.
You were innocent but willingly took the punishment for my crimes.

You beat death and now you stand beside the Father in Heaven preparing me a place at your table.

Hector's kidneys shut down on the eighth day of his hospitalization and dialysis was started. His liver was failing and he had sunk even deeper into coma on the ventilator. His pupils didn't react to light, and he didn't blink, even when the cornea of his eye was stroked with a gauze pad. Neurology ordered an MRI of his brain, which showed multiple injuries in the deep structures of his brain. An EEG showed very slow brain waves.

The nurses had been encouraging me for a few days to talk with Hector's family about code status. They often recognized the threshold of futile care before I did, and they were probably right; Hector's chances of ever waking up were fast approaching zero.

I reported the grave prognosis to Hector's wife and mother and mentioned the comfort care option. The women listened politely, asked a few questions, then expressed that they still wanted aggressive care, making a joint commitment to take Hector home to care for him, even if he remained in a coma for the rest of his life. I was impressed that this didn't require any private discussion between them – they each apparently knew exactly where the other stood. I respected their devotion and didn't try to change their minds. I offered to pray for Hector and they accepted enthusiastically. Hector's nurse Samantha joined us, and we held hands around the bedside, praying together in English (and in Spanish provided by our hospital translator).

Lord Jesus – great doctor!
Nothing is beyond you.
You even brought the dead back to life.
You can heal anything Lord.
We ask you to heal Hector now.
Touch him and make him well.
Let him wake up Lord – be with his wife, his daughter, his mother.

Think of Anabelle Lord – she needs her father!
We cry out to you and we know you hear us.
The Holy Spirit cries out with us.
We will not be put to shame for putting our faith in you!
Raise Hector up. We trust you Lord – we love you. Amen.

Alvarez, our straight-shooting kidney consultant – *and my good friend* – was sitting outside Hector's room at a computer station. He had overheard us and later told me that although he didn't believe in God, he could see how praying with a family would be comforting to them. His comment troubled me for reasons I couldn't immediately put a finger on (as his comments often did). But after some reflection, I silently prayed:

Lord Jesus – don't ever let me pray to you as a "technique" to establish rapport, or to be seen and praised by others.
Let my prayers be <u>sincere</u> and only directed to you, whether in praise or supplication.
If anyone overhears, let it only be to further your designs, not mine.
If anyone is comforted, let it be by your Holy Spirit.

Prayer 229 (August 21, 2021)
How abundant is the goodness that you have in store for those that fear you –that you bestow on those that take refuge in you!
In the shelter of your presence you hide them from all human intrigues.
You hide them safely in your dwelling.
Praise be to the Lord for revealing the wonder of his love!
We were like a people cut off behind enemy lines.
In my alarm I lost sight of you, I called out, and you heard my cry.
Love the Lord all you faithful!
The Lord preserves those that are true to him.
So be strong and take heart, all you who trust in the Lord.
[From Psalm 31]

I went off service, but got a text from Joyce the next day:

"Good morning Anthony. Hector woke up last night and was extubated! I had two long meetings with his family yesterday about his poor prognosis because he was still not waking up or doing anything. Feel a bit of an idiot now, but so happy for him and his family. Heard you prayed for him – ☺ thank you."

I was happy for Hector and his family but shared Joyce's embarrassment about having been so pessimistic. I later realized: Joyce and I were both surprised by Hector's recovery and assumed our shared gloomy attitude was at fault. But this self-blame discounted the possibility that God had answered our prayer – *that Hector's recovery wasn't surprising just because we overestimated how sick he was to begin with, but because a healing miracle had occurred by God's hand.*

Prayer 230 (August 30, 2021)
I recall my purpose today: to praise God and love others.
I know what I should do, but Lord, don't let me forget it.
Don't let me be led astray by trivial distractions.
These can be plainly seen to be from below, because they trigger the emotions of anger, fear and worry.
Jesus has no part in these negative emotions.
Lord, let my mind be calm, rational and at peace.
Let me fear only the Lord, and make my heart a clean dwelling place for your Holy Spirit to abide in.

By late August, we were back up to a double-digit census of Covid pneumonia patients. Two of these, Susan and Mark, were admitted the same day by my partners, although I wouldn't meet either until mid-September. Susan and Mark were ardent Covid deniers, anti–vaxxers, refusing proven therapies and demanding unproven and disproven quackery. This began getting on our nerves and draining our empathy. I'll tell the story of Mark and his family later.

Susan was 44 years old and previously healthy – an ardent anti-masker. When she caught delta Covid, she took ivermectin, zinc and vitamin C. She arrived at our ER about a week later, requiring immediate intubation. Mayfield started standard recommended therapy: dexamethasone and remdesivir, but Susan's husband Connor called in and forbid Susan's nurse from administering the remdesivir*. None of us could ever remember a patient's family restricting our use of an antimicrobial agent for any reason besides a history of an allergic reaction. Family intrusions into critical care management were symptomatic of an unprecedented erosion of trust.

Within a few days of admission, Susan was proned, on 90% oxygen, and receiving a muscle paralysis medication to get her to stop fighting the ventilator. An echocardiogram showed that her heart was severely damaged – another known complication of Covid pneumonia.

Prayer 231 (August 31, 2021)
Oh the depth of the riches and wisdom and knowledge of God!
How unsearchable are his judgments and how inscrutable his ways, or from him, and through him, and to him are all things.
I pray to you for a heart after your heart, not this cruel thing.
Grant me sober judgment – that I should not think of myself too highly, but only according to the measure of faith you have assigned me.
Whatever gifts you have given me, let me exercise them in your service. Let my love be genuine.
Give me the sense to reject evil and hold fast to what is good.
Grant me patience in tribulation, constancy in prayer, generosity in spirit.
Give me your forgiving and merciful heart.
Help me surrender my vengeful spirit and leave it all to your judgment
Lord. Let me not be overcome by evil, but let your Holy Spirit in me overcome evil with good.
[From Romans 11 and 12]

Susan was now on 100% oxygen and multiple pressor infusions to support her severely weakened heart. Her kidneys and liver were failing because her heart wasn't delivering enough oxygen to them. I called Conner to let him know how bad things were going and to emotionally prepare him for Susan's impending death. My first thought was how terrible it was to have to give news like this to him – Connor and Susan were married for over 20 years and had two teenage boys. I asked Conner's permission to be forthright and apologized for being the bearer of bad news. As I laid out the grim tidings, Conner started laughing. I was momentarily stunned – *was I hearing what I thought I was hearing? Maybe he was actually crying. No, he was laughing!*

I interrupted, "I'm sorry Conner, but I don't understand how you could possibly be laughing at what I'm telling you."

"Oh Dr Eckshar, I'm laughing because my wife and I both know that Covid is a hoax. I *know* you're lying to me!"

It was amazing how stubbornly a person can cling to a failing belief system, despite incontrovertible first-hand evidence. But this surreality was becoming routine in our ICU. When that phone call was over, I asked our palliative care team to take responsibility for further communication. Conner later instructed them that "Susan would want everything humanly possible done to prolong her life for the next 100 days" – a request manifestly disjointed from the harsh reality we were facing: Susan wasn't likely to live 100 *hours*, no matter what we did.

Prayer 232 (September 3, 2021)
Consider this statement carefully:
"We know that in all things God works for the good of those who love him, who have been called according to his purpose."
We are those who love him, and we have been called!
[From Romans 8:28-30]

Our ICU service was filling up again with Covid patients. We were up to 31 patients, 14 with Covid pneumonia. I didn't understand how the Delta scourge could be for the good of those that love God, but I *believed* somehow it must. I had given up trying to understand the purpose behind the pandemic anymore. Events would eventually unfold so as to provide some explanation. For now, it was enough to trust God.

Prayer 233 (September 9, 2021)
God, you said, "Let light shine out of darkness!"
You shine in our hearts, to give us knowledge of your glory, reflected in the face of your son Jesus Christ!
Grant that we will not lose heart.
Because although our old bodies are falling apart, you make our spirits new daily.
Don't let hard times bring us down; you use them to prepare us to spend eternity with you.
Help us look away from bad news and focus on your work in the Holy Spirit.
For the things of this world are transient, but our promised home in your kingdom is eternal.
I speak of what I believe, now may our thanksgiving overflow the glory of God.
[An adaptation of 2 Corinthians 4:7-18]

I thought of my physician partners as I wrote this prayer and acted on a feeling I should share it with them. Our group is comprised of members of the Jewish, Jain Dharma, Christian, and Muslim faiths, as well as a few whose faith is unknown to me. It was one thing to share prayer with patients – *but these were my professional business partners.* However, they were also my good friends, and it was likely more than one of them sorely needed encouragement right about now. They responded with unanimous appreciation.

That morning, Susan's O2 sat fell to 15% when she was briefly supined for some nursing care. The nurses re-proned her immediately, barely averting a code arrest. Joyce was on call that evening, and she called Conner to tell him we had to abandon the pretense of full code status. CPR required turning Susan face-up, but her lungs couldn't tolerate that anymore. DNR status was imposed by the reality of the dire situation.

This type of unilateral DNR decision-making, rarely employed pre-pandemic, had now become routine.

Susan died later that night from progressive hypoxemia. I heard that Conner and his sons came into the ICU briefly to be with her, apparently subdued and appreciative. I'm embarrassed to say that I felt sorry for Conner for the first time since he laughed at me, I said a silent prayer for him and his now-motherless boys.

The body of a deceased Covid pneumonia patient in a body bag just before removal to the morgue.

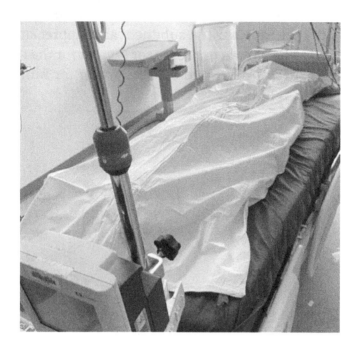

Prayer 234 (September 11, 2021, the 20th anniversary of 911)
It's strange, even though many in our country are letting their Christian heritage fall by the wayside, we are still targeted as a nation of Christians by those who oppose our faith.

Lord, the USA is not your kingdom on Earth, but for the sake our your children here, please bless our country.
Continue to grant us the freedom to worship you.
Comfort those who lost loved ones on 9/11, O Great Comforter!
We know that no material attack can ever put us to shame for putting our faith in you. Lord Jesus, let your name reign on Earth as it does in Heaven and let all knees willingly bend before you.

I stopped down at the grill at 6 am for a breakfast sandwich and coffee. Yuri was there as always. He was making one of our night shift nurses a veggie omelet and toast. She looked tired, her hair a mess – no doubt she had a tough work night. No one else was at the grill counter yet but the three of us. As Yuri handed her breakfast over the stainless steel counter, she started digging around in her purse for her wallet. Yuri scowled, pointing at the exit with his thumb and said, "Psssht!" She looked confused for a second, then smiled, said thanks and headed out. Yuri's perceptive kindheartedness gave me a smile. The hospital was a like a battleship – everyone in the fight together – lifting each other up any we could.

"Hey Yuri – God bless you brother!" He glowered at me and turned back to the grill to finish my sandwich.

Prayer 235 (September 14, 2021)
O my God, in you I trust.
Make me know your ways Lord; teach me your paths.
For you are the author of my salvation.
For your name's sake Lord, pardon my sin, for it is great.
But the friendship of the Lord is for those who fear him.
Turn to me and be merciful – let me not be put to shame for I take
refuge in you!
[Reprise adaptation of Psalm 25]

As mentioned earlier, our patient Mark was admitted in late August. He was unvaccinated despite taking immunosuppressive medications for rheumatoid arthritis. He tested positive for Covid about ten days before admission but refused monoclonal antibody therapy like that taken by President Trump and subsequently proven to reduce hospitalization or death by 80%.

Although it must be pretty obvious to the reader by now that our standard ICU treatments were not highly effective, don't forget by the time patients like Mark arrived in the ICU, they had refused to take prudent precautions to avoid Covid exposure, declined vaccination and rejected the most effective proven treatments available, which must be given *early* in the course of infection. By the time most Covid patients arrived in the ICU, their lungs were already nearly destroyed. This was borne out statistically – the odds of death went up twenty-five times when a patient with Covid was intubated, *not because intubation was harmful*, but because the necessity for intubation indicated how severely their lungs were damaged. The best we could do at this late point was give immunosuppressive drugs like dexamethasone, provide life support and either hope or pray.

Mark's care had been provided by my partners up until now, and his wife and daughter had earned quite a reputation. Like many of our current batch of families, they had some strange theories about Covid treatment that were not exactly our standard practice.

Mark was now on his 22nd hospital day, requiring high-pressure vent settings. His right lung had ruptured and was leaking so badly that almost half of each ventilator breath was coming right back out of his chest tube. *E coli* bacteria were growing out of his sputum, and he experienced repeated episodes of nearly choking to death on purulent secretions, each time requiring emergency bronchoscopy to suction out his airways.

Prayer 236 (September 20, 2021)
Jesus, thanks for two specific gifts of knowledge: knowing that we are among your beloved brothers and sisters, and knowing that how we conduct ourselves in every detail of our life can be used by you to further your kingdom.
These truths give us purpose and hope, from which comes happiness, as can only come through faith in you.
Lord, I dedicate this day to you.
Let the words of my mouth and the intentions of my heart be pleasing in your eyes.

I admit, for the first few days I took care of Mark I purposely avoided his family. But I eventually had to call them, to be sure they understood how badly Mark was doing and to sort out how much longer they thought he would want us to continue life support.

After telephonic preliminaries, Mark's daughter Alex went on the offensive regarding ivermectin. She was very smart and well-read. I could totally understand why she felt that it should be tried, based on what she knew. But there were a few things she didn't know.

Contrary to popular belief, doctors learn some topics in medical school that laypeople, no matter how intelligent, are unlikely to be versed in. Determining the validity of research findings is a science unto itself, involving meticulous review of study methods and in-depth knowledge of potential sources of research error*. It's a very dry topic, and much too complicated to explain to a distraught family member over the phone. I had unsuccessfully tried to explain the fatal flaws of internet-touted ivermectin studies to several other families. I tried a different approach with Alex.

Picking up in the middle of a prolonged and frustrating conversation: "We don't give ivermectin because it hasn't been shown to work." Alex replied, "But why can't we at least *try* it?"

I was getting fed up. "Look Alex. I have to ask you to somehow trust me. I spent four years in med school after finishing college, six more years of internship, residency and fellowship training. I've been in practice for over 35 years. I practice based on my training and experience, not on what Joe Rogan is promoting on Twitter. I'm giving your dad the best care possible – the same treatment I would give my wife Jean if she was in that ICU bed." *I momentarily confirmed the truth of this statement in my conscience.* "I know it's hard to ask you to trust me, but that's what I'm asking from you and your mom. Please trust me to give your dad the best care I can and let me do my job. And by the way, I pray for your dad each day when I see him. I hope that's OK with you and your mom."

"Thanks for praying for him doctor; we have a lot of friends and family praying for him, but we sure would appreciate it if you did too." Alex then posited a theory that turned out to be critical to Mark's ultimate recovery. "But let me just ask you one more thing – is it possible that dad's got *one* good lung now, but the other *bad* lung is what's holding him back?"

"Severe Covid pneumonia always affects *both* lungs Alex," I dismissed her theory to end the interminable phone debate. But that night I lay awake in bed reconsidering her question.

The first thing next morning, I looked carefully at all of Mark's chest X-rays and saw that Alex was on to something – *although I don't understand why she asked that question to this day*. Mark's left lung *had* improved. It was almost imperceivable day by day, but more obvious looking back over a week's worth of X-rays. But the badly-leaking right lung was worsening. I ordered a CT scan that showed the infiltrates typical of Covid pneumonia were clearing, but a large abscess was now occupying a third of Mark's right chest. I discussed Mark's case with one of our thoracic surgeons that morning and he agreed resecting the abscess might restore some function to the remainder of the right lung.

I called Alex and her mother to let them know. Mark was far from being out of the woods, but thanks to Alex's persistent efforts to figure out how to get her Dad home alive, we had a new and more hopeful treatment plan. Our shared faith achieved what no scientific argument could have: it opened my ears to Alex's idea and it opened Alex to trust me.

[*I provide a more detailed definition of critical appraisal of the medical literature in an appendix for the interested reader, but it is only a brief introduction to a complicated topic that I have studied and practiced for years.*]

Prayer 237 (September 25, 2021)
"Shine Jesus shine.
Fill this land with the Father's glory!
Blaze Spirit blaze.
Set our hearts on fire!
Flow river flow.
Flood the nations with grace and mercy!

Send forth your word Lord,
and let there be light!"
[Lyrics by Rich Mullins]

Mark underwent surgery to resect the abscess in his right lung and perform a tracheostomy. Somewhat to the collective amazement of our ICU team, he improved enough within a week to be transferred to a long-term acute care hospital (LTAC), to recuperate and undergo "vent weaning" – the process of coming off the vent and breathing on his own again.

Prayer 238 (October 5, 2021)
Questions I want to ask God about tomorrow:
Will my faith be enough?
Will my eyes be open as your beauty and love are revealed?
Will whatever happens be according to your plan?
Will your grace outweigh my shortcomings?
Will I get a chance to build your kingdom by loving my sisters and brothers?
By the end of the day, will I still be worthy, no matter how badly I might fail?
Will you save me a place by your side in paradise?

Answer: *God does not answer questions in a worldly manner –* saying in the same breath "Yes, yes" and "No, no."
As surely as God is faithful – in the name of the Son of God, Jesus Christ, who conquered death and by whom we are saved through the gift of faith – IT HAS ALWAYS BEEN YES!
[From 2 Corinthians 1:18-19]

We had better-quality isolation gowns during the Delta surge, made of silky yellow polyester. They were laundered after each use and bunches of them were returned to us stuffed in clear plastic bags. Sometimes when you ripped a bag open and pulled a gown out, a tangled bunch would tumble-out *en masse,* necessitating the time-wasting chore of meticulously detangling them and stuffing the extras back into the bag.

After losing my temper with this issue one morning, I had

an idea. I had caught up with my work that morning and could spare a few minutes for recreation. Several nursing co-conspirators and I opened a bag of gowns, pulled out six of them, knotted their sleeves together like a chain of paper dolls, then stuffed them back into the bag. I did all my charting over the next 25 minutes from a computer with line-of-site to that gown bag, waiting to see someone try to pull a single gown out and get all angry when six came out – like a skit on *Candid Camera*. Unfortunately, a "watched pot never boils." To my disappointment, no one used that gown bag during the entire time I sat there. But the goofiness of concocting the prank wasn't entirely wasted; at least it gave us a brief mental reprieve from the suffering and death all around us.

Prayer 239 (October 10, 2021)
As I lay down in bed tonight Lord, I contemplate your greatness.
Creator of all things great and small, your word fills the universe with wonder.
Lover of my soul, who embodied within me a free mind, who gave me my family, everyone I love, and everything I need right down to the air I breathe.
Brave and loving Big-brother, who suffered torture and defeated death to pull me up out of the pit and sanctify me.
There is no other but you. I raise up your holy name.
Let all knees bend and let the Heavens also sing out!
All glory and all honor and all praise to you, Father Son and Spirit abiding in me.
Grant me your peace tonight.

October 2021. Hiking trip with my daughter, Buckskin Gulch, Kane County, Utah.

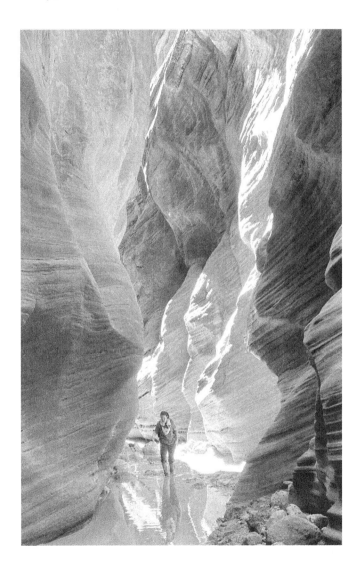

Prayer 240 (October 13, 2021)
Blessed is the one who trusts in the Lord, whose confidence is in him.
They will be like a tree planted by the water that sends out its roots by the stream.
It does not fear when heat comes; its leaves are always green.
It does not worry in a year of drought and never fails to bear fruit.

Lord, all who forsake you will be put to shame, but you are my hope. Search my mind and examine my heart.
Heal me, Lord, and I will be healed; save me and I will be saved, for you alone are the one I praise.
Your glorious throne, exalted from the beginning,
is the place of my sanctuary. [From Jeremiah 17]

We don't take care of sick children in our ICU, but we witnessed some of the pain Covid inflicted on them. Harper was an unvaccinated 37-year-old single mother of three kids aged eight, eleven and seventeen. On admission, she selected her daughter Mia who was "almost eighteen" as her surrogate decision-maker, having no other local family or close friends.

Incredibly, Harper's sister from Nevada, who had been driving to Phoenix to take charge of the children, caught Covid shortly after Harper did. She only made it about halfway to Phoenix before she was overcome by breathlessness, and was admitted to a critical access hospital in Kingman Arizona (where she passed away about a week later). The children now had no other option but to be housed in a shelter during Harper's admission.

Mia's birthday fell on her mom's twentieth ICU day. Harper was comatose on sedation the day Mia officially became her legal surrogate decision-maker, a heartbreaking premature initiation to adulthood. Joyce kindly took Mia under her wing, day by day explaining the situation and helping guide her decisions. Our case worker Sophie stayed in close touch with the kids to be sure they were doing OK in the shelter, typical of her above-and-beyond approach. Mia told Sophie they had all they needed, except for a "vacuum cleaner and shoes." Sophie accessed the funds we collected from our T-shirt sales back in the spring of 2020 and bought backpacks, sneakers, clothes, toys, and a vacuum cleaner, filling the entire trunk of her car and making a delivery to the children at the shelter.

Harper died after a 33-day battle in our ICU. Only thereafter could Sophie help arrange for Mia's grandmother in Mexico to become the legal guardian of the orphaned children. Likely a difficult life ahead for those kids - incredible to think how much sacrifice was now required of them for the lack of the simple precaution of a vaccine shot.

October 12, 2021. *Our kind-hearted case workers Sophie and Jeanette getting a Christmas delivery ready for Harper's three children.*

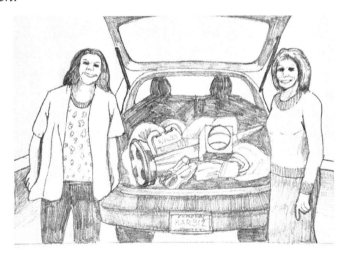

Prayer 241 (October 22, 2021)
Jesus is my shepherd – what else could I ever want?
He has prepared a place for me in Heaven, and he bestows his peace on Earth.
His Holy Spirit keeps me righteous.
No matter what mistakes I make, no matter what earthly

catastrophe befalls, I shall not be afraid because he is with me.
My path is clear.
He lifted me up out of the pit, made strengths of all my
shortcomings and graced me with the highest honor, which even
the angels envy – he called me his son, his brother!
Surely goodness and mercy will follow me all the days of my life
and I will dwell in the house of the Lord forever!
[New Testament version of Psalm 23]

I was working a night shift, had made it through my admissions and into the call room bed by 2 am, tossing fitfully on the cramped single mattress, frequently awoken by pages, but exhausted to the point that I could fall back asleep if given two minutes of peace. At about 4:30 am my pager went off again, but this time as the cobwebs cleared, I realized I could hear a patient screaming from down the hall. I sat up on the side of the bed. My eyelids fel like sandpaper. I had fallen asleep wearing my contact lenses and I blinked a few times trying to loosen them up. A wave of dizziness passed as I took a few deep breaths to get my equilibrium before standing. From the sound of things, I would need to be on full alert.

The screaming was coming from a patient room just a short distance down the hall. I had taken report regarding this patient from the ER doc about an hour earlier and had been waiting for him to arrive in the ICU. His name was Janson, a 27-year-old methamphetamine user with severe agitated delirium and heart failure from methamphetamine-induced cardiomyopathy. Our ICU rooms have large glass sliding doors, so I could see that Janson was being confronted by six or seven nurses as I approached. I estimated he tipped the scales at 270 lbs. He was completely naked, enraged, tottering unsteadily on bare feet and dragging his IV pole behind him tethered by the IV tubing. He appeared both menacing and deathly ill; his face and chest were flushed crimson-red and soaked in sweat; his legs mottled almost purple. The only thing I could think would happen next is that he would fall, splitting his head open on the hard linoleum flood like a watermelon. I imagined trying to catch him if he fell, 270 lbs of naked sweaty dead weight. *I had to get him back in bed.*

Janson was screaming that we had to let him go. He had a right to leave. We didn't have any right to stop him. He was going to leave RIGHT NOW! *Out of his mind; he would die before making it to the elevator.*

I stepped up next to him close range, eye-to-eye.

"Janson. I'm doctor Eckshar. What's the matter?"

"I'm leaving is what's the matter – and THEY ARE TRYING TO STOP ME!"

"OK, OK I hear you. But you're too sick to leave right now."

"Just watch me! I'm LEAVING NOW!"

"Janson, you're too sick." I approached him more closely, and put a hand gently on his shoulder. "You have to stay awhile until you're stronger." He looked suspiciously at my hand, but didn't bat it away. I implored, "Come on brother, let's sit down and talk." He looked me in the eyes, he didn't immediately sit but seemed to calm down a bit. Four able-bodied hospital security guards arrived, but thankfully stood back for now, looking on from the doorway in case needed. Most all the nursing staff that had been in the room when I arrived had now smartly retreated.

"Janson, listen, what can I get you?"

"I'm thirsty, and they won't give me anything to drink" he sulked, his rage momentarily forgotten.

"OK, what do you want to drink? We have ice water – ginger ale?" *For some reason our hospital always seems to have ginger ale on hand.*

"I'm so thirsty – a ginger ale."

I asked the nurses to get us a ginger ale, they looked at me like I was nuts. I probably shouldn't be filling his stomach up with soda if we were going to have to intubate him, but I couldn't renege on him now.

I cajoled Janson to lie back in bed, and he settled down, guzzling his ginger ale. He let me perform a brief bedside echocardiogram. His heart was monstrously enlarged, beating so feebly and rapidly it almost seemed to fluttering. He started getting worked up again. I ordered sedation, but he pulled his IV out using his teeth. His pulse rate steadily rose and his blood pressure began to fall. Unless I could get control of the situation, get him to relax, the acute stress on his badly injured heart was going to kill him. I thought my best option was to heavily sedate and intubate him.

I anticipated that Janson might crash upon receiving sedation for intubation – *blood pressure often bottoms-out when an agitated patient on death's doorstep finally relaxes*. So I had the code cart brought to the bedside and hung a bag of IV Levophed "just in case." The nurses prepared sedation drugs and a neuromuscular blocking agent to completely relax Janson's throat muscles for the intubation. We put him on 100% oxygen through a high-flow nasal cannula to fill his lungs up with as much oxygen as possible – he might need every molecule.

I got around behind his bed, turned the monitor, displaying every heartbeat, blood pressure and O2 sat where I could see it; and positioned a suction wand, ETT and Glidescope* within easy reach.

"OK. Let's go. Give the ketamine and the rocuronium, one, two – now." I kept one eye on the second hand on the wall clock, counting down 45 seconds – *the time it would take the neuromuscular blocking agent to kick in* – my other eye on the rise and fall of Janson's chest, and both ears on the chirp of the audio alarm I had set for his oximeter. The latter would beep for every heartbeat, the musical tone corresponding to his O2 sat, (deepening as it fell).

Thirty seconds – almost there. I glanced at the monitor: blood pressure 85/67 and falling. "Samantha, start that Levophed at 10 mics (10 micrograms per minute)."

Janson's chest rise became subtle then ceased altogether as the neuromuscular blocking agent took effect. The O2 sat immediately began falling, each chirp of the oximeter a lower frequency than the one before in a profoundly disquieting musical progression. *I was going to have to move fast.*

I dropped the head of the bed, scissored his jaws open and inserted the Glidescope down his throat. Janson's pharyngeal anatomy was aberrant – his vocal cords were anterior, difficult to see. The oximeter tone continued to fall ominously. I glanced at the monitor: heart rate 48 and falling – blood pressure 66/35. "Crank that Levophed – 50 mics! Call the code! Samantha – 1 milligram epinephrine STAT."

I adjusted my view, pulling Janson's jaw up with the Glidescope in my left hand and torqued the ETT as far anteriorly as possible – the vocal cords were right there. The tone of the oximeter alarm plummeted alarmingly, but I was within seconds of intubation and I reckoned in that instant that Janson's best chance was for me to complete the intubation rather than back out and try to restore his O2 sat.

Just as the ETT slid through the cords and I inflated the balloon that sealed it in the airway, we lost Janson's pulse. "Start CPR!" Javier coupled his hands over Janson's sternum and started pumping away like an oil well. "Bag him. Bag him!" Sats were in the 60s, 50s. *Was the ETT in the right place?* If I had misplaced it in Jansen's esophagus, he would die now.

But I *hadn't* misplaced it – I was almost certain. I saw it go right through his cords. The O2 sat sometimes initially fell like this right after intubation; it took the heart and lungs a minute or so to pump fresh oxygen out to the tissues where the oximeter resided.

"He's going to come back now that he's tubed," I said aloud – more of a prayer than a prediction. Janson's heart rate on the monitor suddenly jumped to 180! "Hold CPR." I groped his neck searching for the carotid pulse . . . *there!* It was thunderous. The standard code dose of epinephrine we had given – essentially 200 times more adrenaline than the human body releases in a fight-or-flight reaction – was hitting his circulatory system like a freight train, but would only last a minute or two. "Check a blood pressure."

The monitor displayed an O2 sat of 91% and rising, a heart rate of 145 and falling (better). The automatic blood pressure cuff cycled: 148/82. "Sam – start backing down that Levophed slowly." *My* pulse was also falling now.

By the time we were finished, Janson was resting, stabilized on life support, the sun was up, and my night shift was gratefully nearly over.

[*Glidescope is a proprietary flexible fiberoptic videoscope placed over the tongue and down the throat to reveal the vocal cords for intubation.*]

Prayer 242 (October 25, 2021)
In his letter to the Corinthians, Paul said he was called to preach the Good News, but not with wisdom or eloquence, because those would only take away from the cross.
O Lord, you have laid your hand upon me and searched me out.
You know when I lie down and when I rise.
You understand my thoughts before I do and there is not a word on my tongue that you don't know before I speak.
You are always in front, behind, and on both sides of my path and you fashioned my past and my future.
Although it is hard for me to accept, you have taken my guilt away. All my mistakes have been made right by you, and I have been promised a place at the table with you in Heaven for eternity, all on account of the cross.
I sometimes pray for wisdom, for strength or courage, to be a better doctor, but no such attribute I desire could ever change my position with you Lord.
Far, far above anything else I could ever pray for,
I thank you for dying for me and raising me up with you.
Nothing else can compare with that.

I was scheduled to give a talk at a local medical conference on the emotional injury experienced by healthcare workers in a Covid ICU and I asked my friends at work – nurses, case workers, RTs, line team, and everyone else found on the unit that day – if I could take pictures of them to use in my talk.

I noticed something unusual looking through these pictures later as I prepared for the talk. Our team had seen over 800 critically ill Covid patients by this point. Over 350 had died. We had been overworked, stressed-out, vicarious victims of immeasurable anguish, yet the faces of my teammates in the photos conveyed no sense of exhaustion or defeat. Smiling team members stood close together, many with their arms around each other's shoulders or waists. They looked victorious. And I realized *none of us* had overtly burned out during Covid, each individual perhaps realizing that all the rest all depended on them. (I have to add, many of our nurses credited our administrator's great leadership for this abiding sense of team spirit).

The best in some people is elicited by shared adversity. Such teamwork is a beautiful aspect of our God-given nature. *Even Jesus* did not choose to work alone, but surrounded himself with a close circle of people he loved. We were not made to face evil alone – we are so much stronger together.

Prayer 243 (November 1, 2021)
How great you are Father, Son and Holy Spirit.
Your ways are so far above us, we can only begin to understand in the smallest way, your intellect, your cosmic power, and most importantly your love.
We are insignificant, except in your love for us.

I learned something fascinating about God's creation as scientists understand it, having to do with the origin of the atoms that constitute our human bodies. If you include the most common elements that make up organic compounds like carbon and oxygen, elements that are essential to human physiology in small amounts like iodine and copper, and elements that are present in the human body in trace amounts for which there is no currently known physiological purpose, there are 50 different elements present in the human body.

According to astrophysicists, the cosmic origins of those elements are each related to cataclysmic celestial events. Hydrogen was created very soon after the moment of creation in the Big Bang 14 billion years ago – the initial building blocks of all matter. Oxygen was fashioned billions of years later, by the supernovae death–throes of massive stars. Carbon was made when low-mass stars collapsed into super–dense white dwarfs, and when these further imploded into neutron stars, the elements iron and calcium were made. Iodine was made when the densest bodies in all creation, neutron stars, exploded; boron when cosmic rays, emanating from supermassive black holes split the nuclei of larger atoms apart. This is how scientists think God made the fundamental inorganic building blocks of our physical bodies, only the very first preparatory step in the creation of our human selves, which God then endowed with life, a mind, a soul and his love.

How can anyone think this most improbable chain of events could possibly happen without the Creator?

I assume that the things scientists have figured out about creation are accurate for the most part, and basically represent their way of describing God's methods. I respect those who interpret biblical creation more literally than I do, but *if* the scientific explanation of the method of creation is true, it certainly needed simplification back in the days when Genesis was written. We have barely scratched the surface of God's ways even today.

My phone pinged with some good news that afternoon – a text: "Dr. Eckshar, this is Mark's daughter, Alex. I wanted to let you know dad is completely off the ventilator! He is down to 4L of oxygen (about 36% oxygen) through his trach. His body is weak, he is still on a feeding tube, but he has made so much progress in only a few weeks! Thank you so much again for your faith and perseverance. I truly feel God worked his miracle through you!" I texted a reply reminding Alex that it was *her* idea that turned things around for her dad.

Prayer 244 (November 4, 2021)
Where can I go away from your presence?
In Heaven or hell, you would be there.
If I took wing and flew, or dived down to the utmost abyss, even there your right hand would hold me.
If darkness should cover me, the night would be as clear as day, for there is no darkness with you.
Marvelous are your works as my soul well knows.
How I love your Holy Spirit in me!
How great are your councils and blessings –
numbering like the grains of sand in all the world.
I hate those that hate you Lord; your enemies are mine.
I grieve for your lost sheep.
Try me Lord. Seek the ground of my heart.
Prove me and examine my thoughts.
Look well, take any wickedness from me and lead me in your everlasting presence.
And when I wake up tomorrow and go to work again, let it not be with human wisdom or strength, but with your Holy Spirit.
[Reprise adaptation of Psalm 139]

Marg in food services came down the hall rolling her stainless-steel food rack before her. I noticed the rack was full of liter jugs of tube feedings now – only two patient food trays below. Few of our patients were able to eat anymore, most unconscious with feeding tubes snaking down their noses or mouths into their stomachs.

"Hey Marg! Got anything *good* to eat in there? Chocolate ice cream?"

"Hi Doctor! No sorry, no ice cream today!" she smiled, then gestured shyly for me to come closer.

"Doctor – can I ask you something?"

"Sure Marg."

"Do you think I should take the Covid vaccine?" she whispered as though not wanting others to hear.

"Did you ever have a bad reaction to a vaccine?"

"No."

"Then I think you should get it right away Marg. I encourage all my family and friends to get vaccinated as quickly as possible. You see what's been going on here? I don't want to admit you to one of these beds." I shook my finger at her and scowled to get my point across.

"Which one should I get, the Pfizer or the Moderna one?"

"Whichever one you can schedule to get sooner. They are both good."

"OK doctor – I'm going to call CVS when I get home from work today and make an appointment."

As of Nov 2021, we had seen 156 Delta Covid pneumonia patients in our ICU, of whom 152 were unvaccinated. Of the four *vaccinated* patients, three were transplant patients receiving anti-rejection drugs known to severely blunt the immune response to vaccination. The single Covid pneumonia patient who was vaccinated and *not* immunosuppressed did well after one week of mechanical ventilation. So far, seventy of 152 unvaccinated Delta Covid pneumonia patients in our unit had died – seventy husbands, wives, partners, sons and daughters gone. Almost all of them could have been saved by a simple jab.

Prayer 245 (November 9, 2021)
Jesus is the same – yesterday, today and forever – and he has declared: "Never will I leave you; never will I forsake you!"
Therefore, how can mere earthly events harm me?
The Lord is my helper, I will not be afraid.
Lord, grant me contentment with my earthly station.
Bless my family. Strengthen my heart with your grace.
Guide me to follow Jesus and all his saints, especially those that helped me along my way.
Through Jesus, shape my life into an expression of praise, not just in church, but as Jesus did, wherever he was, every minute of every day.

Through your Holy Spirit, let my voice be pleasing to your ears and my actions pleasing in your eyes.
God of peace, who brought back our Lord Jesus from the dead, equip us with everything good for doing your will, and work in us what is pleasing to you, through Jesus Christ, to whom be glory forever and ever.
[From Hebrews 13:5-21]

When I picked up the service this Tuesday morning, I assumed a difficult task. Kent, a 56-year-old man who suffered severe schizophrenia since he was 18 years old, was dying from Covid pneumonia. His mother took care of him from childhood into his mid-thirties, but when she passed away, he was institutionalized. He became hard to control and violent, requiring chronic physical and pharmacological restraints. Food became the primary positive reinforcement for good (=passive) behavior. Now after decades of this treatment, he was chronically bed-bound and completely dependent. Kent weighed 675 lbs. when he was admitted to our ICU.

Over his three-week ICU admission, Kent followed a progressive downhill course of mechanical ventilation like many previously described. Given his dismal outlook for survival, poor quality of life, and lack of any surviving family or friends, Mayfield had petitioned a court to establish DNR status and transition Kent to comfort care. This request was granted yesterday, on Mayfield's last day on service, and now my job was to help Kent die in peace with as little suffering as possible.

I talked to Kent's nurse Lynn about the medications to administer in case Kent experienced pain or breathlessness. She agreed, observing, "It's sad Kent doesn't have anyone to be with him today." I figured that was her way of inviting me to hang out with them awhile after we pulled the tube.

Right after lunch, we went ahead. We started with initial moderate doses of morphine and lorazepam (an anti-anxiety medication) which would not suppress Kent's respiration but would help keep him from being scared or short-of-breath when we pulled the tube. (We never give comfort care medications to hasten or bring about death, only to ameliorate suffering, and studies have shown that patients on comfort care live longer when they receive such medications.)

We extubated Kent, and he seemed apathetic as he breathed natural air for the first time in three weeks. His breathing wasn't labored, but his O2 sats began steadily falling. Kent's eyelashes were glued shut with crusted secretions. Lynn gently cleaned them with a warm washcloth. Kent opened his eyes and stared mutely at the ceiling with no discernable emotion. He hadn't been shaved in a while, and I noticed some debris in his beard. His vast and misshapen corpus, constrained between the bedrails, bespoke an unfathomable history – *how could this have been allowed to happen?* But if you tried, you could still imagine the young man Kent once must have been, the forgotten hopes his mother must have once had for him . . .

Lynn and I watched silently for any sign of distress requiring further palliation, as other folks from the unit trickled into the room: Sophie, Isaiah, Sam, Javier (who had placed Kent's IVs). Most lightly touched Kent somewhere – his foot, his hand. Sophie started telling him all about her recent vacation trip to Myrtle Beach in a soft familiar voice, like they were old friends, describing the warm sand under her bare feet, how good it felt wadding into the calm blue waters. While she calmly intoned, her hand snuck up to Kent's shoulder (as if she hoped no one would notice) and began gently stroking it in a comforting gesture, such as his mother might provide if she were present.

My reverie stumbled momentarily – *had Kent ever seen a beach?*

I looked at his face, considered his institutionalized life – prayed there was some period of happiness, some chance that Sophie's story could transport him back to a pleasant memory from his childhood. All in all, about a dozen of the ICU staff visited Kent during the two hours during which he slowly passed away – filling in for family and friends he didn't have.

Prayer 246 (November 15, 2021)
Sometimes I forget, but we are your chosen people, a royal priesthood, a holy nation, your special possession.
We declare your praises for calling us out of the darkness into your wonderful light.
Once we were scattered, alone and lost.
But now you have gathered us together, called us "The People of God."
Once we were guilty and justly sentenced to death, but you have granted us mercy – taken us out of the jail, washed us, arraigned us in clean clothes, and seated us in the place of highest honor.
You bore our sins in your body on the cross; by your wounds we were healed.
For we were like stray sheep, but now returned to the Shepherd and the Keeper of our souls.
[Adaptation of 1 Peter 2:9-24]

Prayer 247 (November 19, 2021)
I thank him who has given me strength – Christ Jesus our Lord – because he judged me faithful, appointing me to his service, although formerly I was his prideful enemy.
I received mercy because I acted in ignorance and unbelief and the grace of our Lord overflowed for me with the faith and love that are in Christ Jesus.
The saying is trustworthy and deserving of full acceptance that Christ Jesus came into the world to save sinners, of whom I am the foremost.
But I received mercy so that Jesus Christ could display his perfect patience, even for one such as me, as an example to those who were to believe in him for eternal life.
Now my destiny is no longer determined by sin and filled with the gift of his Holy Spirit, I am pleasing in his sight.
To the King of the ages: the only God, be honor and glory forever

and ever.
[From 1 Timothy 1:12-17]

We had 27 patients on our census that week. Nine were unvaccinated Covid pneumonia patients, five of whom were on what would turn out to be a fatal downhill course. Yet some of our sickest were non-Covid patients:

A homeless 58-year-old methamphetamine user found unconscious in the street, in septic shock, his back and legs covered with infected pressure ulcers.

A 29-year-old woman with a familial clotting system disorder who suffered a massive stroke destroying the entire left side of her brain.

A 63-year-old man on a ventilator in a prolonged coma from West Nile Virus acquired by a mosquito bite.

A 24-year-old man with advanced AIDS and fungal pneumonia who weighed 89 pounds*.

An 82-year-old man with squamous cell cancer invading his left eyeball and brain, allowing air to enter into his skull (a rare and horrible condition called "pneumoencephaly"). He was full code despite his dismal prognosis.

A 27-year-old man on a ventilator after he overdosed on M30 street fentanyl and aspirated vomit into his lungs.

A 25-year-old female narcotic user who underwent surgery for an infection in her jaw. She was in tremendous pain – her mouth wired-shut with a stainless steel fixation device. Tolerant to the action of painkillers because of her chronic daily use, she wailed continuously and inconsolably no matter how much narcotics we administered. Her incessant anguished cries, according to Mayfield, were like "a background soundtrack from hell."

[*I was a medical student in the early 80s when AIDS emerged. Back then, AIDS patients with fungal "pneumocystis" pneumonia who required intubation invariably died. Now, almost forty years later, I had more optimism for my patient with advanced AIDS than I had for our intubated Covid pneumonia patients. He had a better chance of making it out of the unit alive – and he eventually did.]*

Prayer 248 (November 22, 2021)
Lord, I feel like under attack today.
So many disappointments and setbacks – things that should have been easy to accomplish became nearly impossible.
I'm driven to swear in frustration.
Help me see these for what they are – attacks on my spirit.
Don't let me fall for it.
Because Satan would have me defile my own soul, make it an unfit dwelling for your Holy Spirit.
Satan has some power over me while I'm on Earth, but he can't make me do anything without deceiving me into going along with him. Armor-plate my soul against his attack.
If I keep my eyes on yours Lord, there is nothing he can do to harm me. [See Ephesians 6:10-18]

It was late in another mind-numbing work shift when I got a call from the ER about a possible ICU admission – *my seventh new admission of the day*: a 59-year-old man with Covid pneumonia named Clifford. He had mild pneumonia on his chest X-ray, a normal blood pressure, and only required standard low-flow nasal oxygen. We wouldn't normally consider ICU admission for such a patient, but the ER doc had noticed some enlarged lymph nodes in Cliff's neck suggesting the possibility of underlying systemic disease, possibly cancer. This was of immediate concern because it indicated his immune system might be dysfunctional. I recommended admission to a regular hospital bed at first, but changed my mind after thinking about it. I called the ER back and accepted Cliff's admission to our ICU.

He came up from ER to the unit at 6:30 pm, right near the end of my shift – was sitting up in his ICU bed texting friends when I walked in the room, introduced myself and briefly touched base with his nurse. I could tell the nurse didn't quite approve of admitting a patient that looked so well to the unit. I took Cliff's history, examined him – *those lymph nodes were definitely significant, not only in his neck but in his armpits and groin; they would have to eventually be biopsied* – and left the room to write my note and enter orders. The later included our standard Covid therapy: dexamethasone (proven to reduce Covid mortality) and remdesivir (less convincingly shown to reduce the duration of Covid). We don't normally give antibiotics to a patient admitted with Covid since antibiotics don't work on viruses and it had been shown that Covid patients rarely had secondary bacterial infections at the time of admission. But I decided to order two of our strongest antibiotics, piperacillin/tazobactam and vancomycin STAT, just in case Cliff's immune system was weakened by whatever was residing in those lymph nodes.

Prayer 249 (November 23, 2021)
[This was an unshared personal prayer]
I made a fatal mistake yesterday at work Lord.
You know it was my mind and not my heart that failed, but a patient suffered a terrible consequence.
Bless the man I harmed Lord – I pray he is with you now.
Lift this burden from me, which my conscience cannot bear.

The next morning, I got to the hospital at about 6 am and stopped by the cafeteria to grab breakfast, asking Yuri to make me "the usual". While waiting in line at the grill I bumped into one of the night shift ICU nurses who confided to me they had a terrible night. The Covid patient I admitted had rapidly deteriorated after I went home for the night, coded and died.

Cliff had died. *What had I missed?*

I scarfed down my sandwich and coffee without any appetite *but knowing I would need fuel*, and hurried up to the unit to find Mayfield. He related the events of the evening.

Cliff was already rapidly decompensating when Mayfield saw him at the beginning of his shift, spiking a fever of

104° and lapsing into delirium. Mayfield started antibiotics, but Cliff declined meteorically – completely "whiting-out" both lungs over four hours! (*Lungs that are completely filled with pus become white on chest X-rays*)

Mayfield intubated Cliff, but by 4 am it became impossible to oxygenate him or to maintain his blood pressure despite four pressors. Cliff passed away despite full life support. At 5 am, Cliff's blood cultures grew a virulent bacteria – *Klebsiella pneumoniae*. He died from septic shock due to simultaneous infection by two life-threatening pathogens present upon admission: Covid and Klebsiella.

But one detail of the story puzzled me – Mayfield said *he* started antibiotics at the beginning of his shift. I had already started Cliff on antibiotics at the end of my shift, almost an hour earlier. I signed onto the EMR and checked. There was no computer entry showing I had ordered antibiotics. I checked "current orders," "order history" and "medication history." Nothing. I called the pharmacy and asked them to check. There was no record that I ordered antibiotics.

I *had* decided to give antibiotics, documented the plan in my note, and would have sworn that I had entered the orders in the computer, but somehow I had failed to complete the task. There was no telling whether getting antibiotics an hour earlier would have saved Cliff's life, but it was impossible not to obsess over that possibility. My lapse might have been the final nail in Cliff's coffin.

I lost many subsequent nights of sleep trying to understand my mistake. Our complicated computer physician order entry system certainly played a role. I went back later and counted eight steps in the process required to complete an electronic antibiotic order. An interruption anywhere along the process could derail the whole thing – an urgent page, a tap on the shoulder by a nurse with a question – I couldn't remember how I lost track of what I was doing. Another factor was bad timing. My failed order-entry came right at the end of a 12-hour shift, so I never had a second chance to catch my mistake and fix it. (Thankfully, Mayfield came along right behind me to catch it.) But regardless of *how* it happened, the responsibility was still all mine.

For months afterward, whenever I entered routine orders for a patient, I thought about how relatively trivial these were compared to Cliff's antibiotic orders. That's one hard thing about the unit – a simple mistake at just the wrong moment can have unforgettable tragic consequences. I retain a vivid memory of the last time I saw Cliff, sitting in his ICU bed, texting his friends and family – none of us aware this would be his last day on Earth.

Prayer 250 (November 24, 2021)
Out of the deep have I called unto you, O Lord – hear my plea.
If you kept a record of sins Lord, who could stand?
But you are merciful so that we can serve you with reverence.
I wait for you Lord with my whole being – like a watchman in the
night. In your word I put my hope!
Your unfailing love Lord is the source of my redemption!
[From Psalm 130]

As I rounded in the ICU this morning, exhausted by last night's grinding insomnia and perhaps dangerously preoccupied with Cliff's death, I received another text from Alex: "Dr. Eckshar. Parent update: Dad has been off the ventilator completely now for more than two weeks. The feeding tube has been removed, and he is eating meals and drinking water, coffee, milk, and Sprite. He walked 50 feet yesterday and is gaining strength every day with physical therapy. Dad is texting now and using the speaking valve all day. This Thanksgiving, I am so thankful for the miracle God has given my family and for you, Dr. Eckshar. You and the nurses saved my dad's life."

This text was like a life preserver thrown to me as I drowned. Thank God I had shared my cell phone number with Alex.

Prayer 251 (November 28, 2021)

Many times Lord, I prayed for you to take away my failings.
But you said "My grace is sufficient for you Anthony, for my power is made perfect in your weakness."
You told me to accept my limitations and let Christ's power rest in me. Help me learn that truth.
Jesus, for your name's sake, help me accept my internal shortcomings and external hardships, because when I am too weak, your spirit in me is always strong enough to overcome!
[From 2 Corinthians 12]

Back when Dom and I worked together in the ICU, I could rely on him to debrief me after I made any serious medical mistake, whether or not it led to patient injury. He would ask me to stop by his office to talk a few days later, in the afternoon after things had quieted down. He'd sit down and look expectantly at me from across his desk (always covered with neat piles of medical journals) waiting for me to speak first. I'd explain what happened, what I did wrong and why, what I wished I had done and what I would do *next time*. Once I got it all out of my system, Dom would pass merciful judgment, reassuring me that I was still OK. *Mr.* Eckshar, (making fun of the fact that someone like me could end up being a doctor), the most important thing is that you care." Having big brother to share my mistakes with was one of the things I missed most about Dom.

Over 30 years of practice together, I was privy to the realization that even *Dom* made serious mistakes. Knowing that my hero was fallible helped me forgive my own shortcomings.

Dom's judgment regarding errors was based on our shared philosophy: "A good doctor can be trusted to always place his/her patient's best interest first, with ability, good judgment, and a caring attitude." Errors that occur *despite this approach* are inevitable and forgivable, but never forgotten *–this is how* *we learn not to repeat them.* This philosophy helped us deal with our mistakes intellectually, but it didn't entirely protect our spirits.

The final event that caused Dom's eventual burnout was not really a mistake but rather a tragic consequence of a judgment call he made. He gave an unapproved blood-clotting medication to a young lady with life-threatening postpartum hemorrhage (internal bleeding associated with childbirth) after all other measures had failed. The patient survived but suffered a disabling stroke due to excessive blood clotting. The physician "peer-review" committee (comprised of doctors who primarily practiced in the office) classified his actions as "substandard care causing serious patient injury". At the point Dom was in his career, this was a crushing indictment. I don't know how many honest "errors" such a good doctor's conscience can bear. But each one leaves a scar and the more you care, the deeper it goes.

The obstetrical stroke case was perhaps the final slash in Dom's "death by a thousand cuts." Shortly thereafter, in the fall of 2013, Dom reached the point where he just couldn't take it anymore. He had shared in the suffering of his patients, been held responsible for catastrophic events largely outside his imperfect human control too many times. We didn't know the term back then, but Dom met all the diagnostic criteria of what is now called burnout, *except for one:* he never suffered compassion fatigue. He cared about his patients and their families until the end. But over time, even that wasn't enough to keep his head above water. He announced his premature retirement to the group and we lost the best ICU doctor any of us knew.

Dom later warned me: "Anthony, be careful. Whatever happened to me could happen to you someday. Don't be too hard on yourself. Spend time with your family. Focus on being happy. You're ten years behind me – don't follow me down this road."

Since then, I tried to follow Dom's advice. I leaned into my faith and the love of my family. Although not often mentioned in these stories, Jean was secretly part of every one. She listened to my daily reports – every high and low. She consoled, celebrated and encouraged me; prayed for my patients every night. Jean healed me up each evening so that I could go back to the ICU again the next morning. In her, I had one saving grace that Dom never had. So, although the thought I might be burning out crossed my mind, it wasn't for long. I was acutely aware of my exhaustion, my obvious fallibility, but that just meant I had to be even more careful. Anyway, I couldn't be spared. If I burned out now, who was going to take my place? This wasn't any special virtue on my part, I was pretty sure my ICU family all felt the same way.

Prayer 252 (December 5, 2021)
Lord Jesus, my purpose in life ought to be to obey you, and your purpose is to glorify the Father and serve the undeserving.
What a beacon of love you are Lord, in a dark and stormy sea!
Let my life have eternal purpose Lord – let me follow in the path you have blazed.

We admitted an unvaccinated 32-year-old man who went by his initials: "PJ." He was intubated in the ER for Covid pneumonia and unconscious the entire time I took care of him. PJ had the image of a rosary tattooed around his neck, a solid black Spanish-style cross, eight inches tall, emblazoned across his sternum. That much ink must have *hurt*, so although I never once spoke with PJ, I knew something personal about him.

Later the same day, we admitted an unvaccinated 60-year-old cattle rancher named Carter. Carter's family lived in a remote rural area of northeastern Arizona where it didn't seem like Covid vaccination was necessary they had so little interaction with outsiders. More about PJ and Carter later. I had plenty of other Covid patients to keep me busy for the time being.

As Mayfield and I were sitting next to each other

on the unit doing some charting, *Hark the Herold Angels Sing* was streaming in the background. Two patients were simultaneously screaming from rooms down the hall. One man, bedbound and robbed of coherent speech by a stroke, was incessantly moaning in a high-pitched warble. The other, a delirious alcoholic who had been in a major motor vehicle accident, was crying out: "Help me, help me, help me, help me, help me," no matter how many times the nurses went into the room to attend to him. The contrast between the music and the patients' apparent unremitting torment was otherworldly. "I feel like I'm in purgatory," said Mayfield. "I can hear Heaven and hell at the same time from here."

Prayer 253 (December 9, 2021)
*Jesus, I'm having a hard time figuring out what I need to do
to draw closer to you.*
*Not good works – you have given me opportunities to do good works
for my benefit, not yours.*
*Not avoiding sin – my sins don't matter any more thanks to your
perfect sacrifice on my behalf.*
*Not somehow hiking-up my own faith – you give me faith in the
measure and timing that I require.*
*Not making myself holy – I failed at that, yet you filled me with
your Holy Spirit.*
The only thing I think I need to do is to seek you.

*I seek you Lord, in the morning when challenges lay ahead and in
the night when my successes and failures lay behind.*
I seek your aid in adversity.
I seek your presence when I feel empty and alone.
I seek your counsel and blessing in difficult decisions.
I seek your beauty in the sky, in the seashore, plants and animals.
I seek to understand the majesty of your creation.
*I seek you in the kindness of strangers, and the love of close friends
and family.*
*I know now: I will never feel close enough to you while I'm here on
Earth; all I can do now is continue to seek you until I am by your*

side in Heaven.

While our unit was overrun with unvaccinated Covid pneumonia patients – *the beds of those who died immediately filled by others waiting in the state triage system* – outside the hospital, it was business as usual. Few people were wearing masks in stores or restaurants; every bar and gym was open for business. Our state government was either incapable or unwilling to encourage social distancing. Our federal government had lost the information battle. If you just looked around the city outside the ICU, it would appear as though hundreds of thousands of Americans were *not* dying from Covid – *what other logic could explain our collective passivity?* It felt like I was living in two completely different worlds, parallel universes with separate realities: one focused on a grim battle with suffering and death, the other on denial.

Prayer 254 (December 12, 2021)
Lord God, Father – do not turn your face away.
Used to be, you could do that.
But now, by your Son's sacrifice, you cannot despise those of us whom you have chosen and whom your Son died to save.
We are innocent by his blood.
Save us from lies, fear and our stubborn pride.
Covid is turning us against each other Lord.
Shower your love down on the Earth through us.
Take away division and distrust; nurture us and unite us as your children.

We had been taking care of a married couple in their mid-40s now for over two weeks – Roz and Aaron. They owned a high-adventure outdoor recreation business, didn't have any kids, but ran a charitable outreach program enabling handicapped children to participate in activities like hiking and skiing. Roz and Aaron caught Covid after attending a crowded recreational gear convention in Las Vegas, unmasked and unvaccinated. This was the first time I ever requested

ECMO for a husband and wife simultaneously; they were both turned down because all ECMO programs in the city were at capacity. They had been racing each other toward the ultimate finish line and both died today, within six hours of each other.

In other cases on our service, relatives of dying patients refused standard therapies but requested apple cider vinegar, inhaled hydrogen peroxide, and colloidal silver – folk remedies with no rational scientific basis and unknown safety. "Just trying them" based on desperation was insupportable in my mind, an abandonment of the evidence-based practice of medicine that I built my entire career upon.

A wife whose husband was dying from Covid in our ICU confided in me something that her husband <u>could never find out</u>, that she had secretly been vaccinated – *as though this was the worse thing she could have done.* Another woman who called Covid "fake news" experienced a highly fatal outbreak at her family-owned business where no one was vaccinated or wore masks. Her brother and husband both died from Covid. She initially refused to have her husband buried in an attempt to coerce the treating physician into taking Covid off the death certificate.

Yet, although the material belief system of these patients and their families was opposed to all my training and experience, their spiritual belief system was akin to my own. God had put me in the position to relate to, forgive, educate, and love them. Our Christian family ties might just be the one thing that could overcome the ideological contention that had us at each other's throats.

Prayer 255 (December 16, 2021)
I am personally speechless – taking a break to sit and listen to what the Holy Spirit has to say.
The word of God, embodied in Jesus Christ, who through his sacrifice now lives in my soul, is always ready to speak if I will only take a minute out of my busy day to listen.
I now listen . . .

God says to me, "I am. I made you."
"I love you, but you were made to do my will, not yours.
You have no choice but to endure adversity, but you can choose
how to endure it: with faith in your loving Father, sure knowledge
that you are returning to his home forever someday soon, forgiving
your brothers and sisters whatever they do, and in turn being
forgiven, or just surviving without a clear purpose, waiting for the
nothingness of death, stubbornly clinging to resentment, pride and
fear."

You have opened my eyes again today Lord.
How can I pick the path of destruction when you have made a clear
way for me to return home to you?
I chose your way again today Lord.
Help me every day as I stumble, though the path you offer is wide
and straight. I couldn't go one step down it if not for you!

Mark had his feeding tube and tracheostomy removed and made it home to his wife Clare today, on their 36th wedding anniversary – their daughter Alex celebrating with them.

Almost to the day of the first anniversary of my first Covid vaccine, Arizona's Governor Ducey issued an executive order <u>prohibiting</u> any county, city or town in Arizona from issuing a Covid vaccine mandate. Firm evidence would later show that the vast majority of the Delta and Omicron deaths we had witnessed could have been prevented by vaccination.

Prayer 256 (December 19, 2021)
Jesus, let me eat and drink and enjoy whatever labor is allotted to me by the Father today.
Remind me not to worry and to be thankful for whatever happens next, because everything proceeds according to your plan, and you are saving me a seat at your table when my work here is done.
[Taken from Ecclesiastes 2:24-25]

The Omicron Covid variant, identified in Botswana, S.

Africa, in November 2021, arrived in the United States by December and was causing the incidence of Covid to skyrocket again. Just as Delta was twice as infectious as earlier strains of Covid, Omicron was twice as infectious as Delta. There was little respite between the Delta and Omicron surges; they merged into the most prolonged surge of the pandemic. It was starting to look as though Covid could mutate faster than our natural immunity and vaccine science could keep up.

Now, I considered the dreadful prospect of another Christmas spent in the Covid ICU. There was a palpable discordance between the expected merriment of the season and the surging mortality of our patients, that I don't think I will ever to able to mentally detangle. I wrote these Christmas carol lyrics during a boring stretch in the early hours of a sleepless night shift and posted them in our call room, perhaps as an expression of the grim and paradoxical association between Covid and Christmas. As the saying goes, "Sometimes laughing is the only thing that can keep you from crying."

Sung to the tune of "I Saw Mommy Kissing Santa Claus"
I saw Mayfield tubing Santa Claus
From behind his P100 mask.
He didn't see me creep
To the vent to up the PEEP*
He thought I had collapsed in the call room in a heap!

Then I saw Mayfield bronching Santa Claus.
Sucking out secretions snowy-white
Oh what a code it would have been
If he had left that sputum in
And just let him take iver-mectin!
[*PEEP is a pressure setting on the vent]

Prayer 257 (December 22, 2021)
Oh that you would rend the Heavens and come down, that the mountains would tremble before you and you would make your name known to your enemies.

Since ancient times, no one has perceived, no ear has heard, no eye has seen any God besides you – who acts on behalf of those who wait for him.
You come to the aid of those who gladly do right in your name, who remember your ways.
Do not remember our sins Lord, for the sake of your Son's blood.
Look on us with mercy, for we are your people!
[Based on Isaiah 64]

Christmas was just a few days away, but I felt no holiday spirit. Yet I felt guilty that I hadn't done any decorating at home. After work, I pulled our stale-smelling artificial tree out of a dusty box in the garage and put it up, showering detached needles all over the great room floor. I found one tangled string of lights that still worked. When I was done, the tree reminded me of the one from *Charlie Brown Christmas* before Linus fixed it up with his blanket.

Prayer 258 (December 25, 2021, Christmas Day)
Jesus, what a leap of faith it was for you to set aside your omnipotence and take the form of a helpless infant in a savage and primitive environment; starting life as a refugee in a distant land; fleeing the threat of execution.
The first of your human miracles showed us how completely you were committed to our salvation.
We thank you and praise your holy name this Christmas day!

I should mention that I had honored my commitment to pray with every patient every day throughout this surge (and did so right up until the Covid ICU nightmare finally ended). The service was very busy over Christmas weekend.

Among almost 20 other patients, I picked up care of Carter, the 60-year-old cattle rancher with Covid pneumonia admitted a few weeks previously. Carter was receiving 70% oxygen by mechanical ventilator and slowly worsening. I was too busy to communicate much with his family, but I laid my hands on and prayed for Carter every day.

PJ was deteriorating on maximal ventilator settings. He was intolerant of proning; it made his O2 sat *fall* from the 80s into the 70s when it was attempted. He was turned down for ECMO. We tried an inhaled medication called epoprostenol – a last-ditch attempt to boost O2 sat when all other methods failed, but it had only equivocal benefit. Each day, the huge cross tattooed on PJ's chest reminded me to pray the Lord's Prayer out loud in PJ's room.

On Christmas Eve, Mayfield and I talked it over and made PJ a "two-doc DNR." As previously mentioned, establishing DNR status in the pre-pandemic era involved shared decision-making with patients or their families. But some of our Covid patients were so sick that coding them had no chance of providing any benefit. We were too busy now to debate such cases. PJ was already on the highest levels of life support we could provide; if that wasn't enough, we didn't have anything left to offer. If PJ's heart stopped, he was done.

Although this decision was made unilaterally, I needed to at least inform PJ's family. But I put it off calling them, having already conveyed all the bad news I could stomach that day. But on Christmas day, I had a free minute about mid-afternoon and I looked up PJ's family contact in our EMR; it was his grandfather, *also named PJ*.

I froze, staring at his phone number on the computer screen. It didn't feel like Christmas here in the ICU, *but it was Christmas outside.* How could I call Grandpa PJ on Christmas day to tell him his grandson was going to die?

I couldn't.

And if I couldn't reveal the DNR order, I couldn't honestly abide by it either. I rescinded it and made PJ full code again. I can't rationally defend my decision-making process, and I sometimes wonder if I would have thought differently if it weren't Christmas day or if PJ wasn't named after his grandpa. But that's what happened. PJ survived Christmas day and over the next few weeks, slowly began to recover.

Prayer 259 (December 28, 2021)

Lord Jesus – thank you for opening your arms to a stubborn and foolish people.

Thank you for forgiving our shortcomings and calling us your brothers and sisters – children together of your great and loving Father. Grant us unity. Grant us your peace.

I praise you for the rebirth of prayer I see in the families of our patients – your lifeboat for us in the stormy sea.

Just like in the olden days Lord, you shelter those you have chosen to gather at your feet in the midst of catastrophe.

No matter what Earthy adversity comes next, we can overcome anything if you stand over us.

My ICU shift started with unacceptable efficiency, the kind that could later lead to errors of omission. I looked at the time – 8:43 am. I had been working for over two-and-a-half hours and had seen only two patients. I had fifteen more on my list, would also have to cover another fifteen once Joyce checked out, and could get three more admits before the capacity of the nursing staff was completely saturated – *more* if any of our patients died. Each death opened a bed to yet another Covid patient awaiting admission.

I pulled up a new patient's chart on the computer and started trying to make sense of it: A 42-year-old woman admitted with two separate, simultaneous hemorrhagic strokes. She had no history of high blood pressure, diabetes or heart disease and wasn't on any blood thinners. *That didn't make sense – how does someone get two strokes at the same time with no risk factors?* I was missing something – something potentially life-threatening. *She had a history of melanoma – could the "strokes" actually be brain metastases?* My pager went off: the transfer center with another admit. A nurse walked up, standing behind me as I took the call, not wanting to interrupt, but hovering just within my personal space until she had a chance to catch my eye. A consulting physician also walked up more directly into my field of vision – I had to tell them that I was on the phone although it was obvious since I was holding the phone receiver to my ear.

As soon as I got off the phone, I spoke to the nurse and doctor, then looked back at the computer monitor. *Where was I?* The woman with two strokes had a fever of 101.5. *Could the so-called strokes represent a bloodborne infection spreading to the brain? Endocarditis – an infection of her heart valves? I should re-examine her heart, do an echo, order blood cultures, and antibiotics.* I started entering orders just as another nurse interrupted to ask me for Tylenol for her patient having a headache, to which I assented without even looking up. I tried to get back to entering the antibiotic orders but my pager went off again – the ER. *They could wait.* I looked up the antibiotic dosing in Up-to-date online. As I entered the orders for antibiotics, I wondered if I should perform a lumbar puncture – *would that be safe given the pressure the hemorrhage was putting on her brain?* I needed to curbside (unofficially consult) our neurosurgeon for an opinion on that. But before I could text them, another nurse came up, "Room 364's family is on the phone. They're mad, demanding to talk to a doctor."

I snapped. "Listen! I can't talk to them right now OK? I have to figure out what's wrong with this lady!" pointing at the computer screen as though it were a person. "But *I can't do that* if I keep getting interrupted every ten seconds!" I stormed out of the ICU and into our call room, slamming the door behind me and making myself temporarily inaccessible. I took some deep breaths and concentrated on the woman with two strokes long enough without interruption to formulate a plan, enter all her orders, and make absolutely sure the antibiotic orders went through. Then I sequentially answered three pages received in the interim.

One of the pages was the ER in regards to a patient named Salvatore, who was "found down" at home. When EMS responded, they found the patient in "asystole" – the medical term used when the heart's electrical activity completely ceases. Asystole is essentially indistinguishable from death itself, except that when it first occurs there is still a slight chance that the patient might be resuscitated with rapid intervention. But ACLS initially failed to restore a heartbeat, and our ER physician instructed EMS to cease resuscitation and declare the patient dead in transit. EMS inexplicably disregarded this order and delivered the patient to our ER where our staff continued ACLS for another 35 minutes. At this point, Salvatore's heart finally resumed electrical activity with the assistance of numerous life-support drugs and a mechanical ventilator.

I brought up Salvatore's medical record and learned that he was known to have terminal lung cancer with metastases to his liver and spine. I added up a cumulative CPR duration of 65 minutes! The chances he would ever awaken, or even survive the next few hours, were as close to zero as anything in medicine. The ER was now requesting that I admit Salvatore to the ICU, as though prolonging his death process as long as possible was a reasonable shared goal. And I had no choice but to accept.

Salvatore appeared clinically brain dead on arrival in the ICU, a diagnosis which was confirmed by a brain perfusion study that showed absolutely no blood flow to his brain. I prayed for his soul awkwardly, not sure how it worked – *praying for a dead person.* I imagined him with Jesus' arm around his shoulder. I called his son, who was actually somewhat relieved that "Sal" had passed; he had greatly suffered and the family was aware that his end was near. "He never would have wanted to get CPR."

After I completed all the associated paperwork associated with Salvatore's death, I called the ER doc and asked *why* he would code a patient with terminal lung cancer for 65 minutes. (Code efforts are typically discontinued after 20-25 minutes if the patient doesn't respond, shorter in patients with asystole, who survive to discharge in less than 1% of cases.) Sixty-five minutes of code effort is extraordinarily unusual. The ER doc couldn't give me any rational explanation. Perhaps the thought that he could have "called the code" had never crossed his mind. At least he seemed mildly chagrined; I guessed that's all I could hope for.

I heard someone once say the main qualification for becoming a doctor was "the courage to bear witness to death." If so, it was a qualification none of us wanted to exercise. Some patients were sent to the ICU only because it is a convenient location to die. In hopeless situations, it's easier for almost every other kind of doctor to "kick the can down the road" but those of us in the ICU resided at the end of the road. We were thereby destined to bear witness to nearly every single patient's death.

Prayer 260 (December 29, 2021)
Lord – You have said to me: "Fear not, for I have redeemed you. I have summoned you by name Anthony; you are mine."

When I pass through raging rapids, you are with me.
When I pass through fire, I will not be burned.
You have called me precious and honored in your sight, and because you love me, you have ransomed my soul by your holy blood. You have given me back new life.
I will not be afraid, for you are with me.
You will call your children together from the four corners of the Earth – every son and daughter created for your glory.
You have called us each by name and we will stand together as your witnesses to all the nations of the world.
Your holy scriptures have foretold all that has happened.
It is true! We know and believe.
Before you, there was nothing, nor will there be anything after you. Apart from you, there is no other savior.
YOU ALONE ARE GOD, now and forevermore!
[Modern interpretation of Isaiah 43, part 1]

Thirty-four of our 36 ICU patients had Covid pneumonia. The unit looked like a war zone – the hallways an obstacle course of IV infusion pumps, ventilator control panels, racks of PPE, clean plastic-wrapped proning beds awaiting new occupants. One patient had so many IV infusion pumps that the nurses had been able to arrange them roughly into the shape of a Christmas tree on the overloaded chrome IV pole outside his room – the red and green indicator LEDs like a string of blinking Christmas lights.

A third of my patients died over the three-day weekend. I barely noticed how horrible that was until after I had been off a day and was able to reflect. I was getting numb to death. Carter was among those who looked like they weren't going to make it. The palliative care team met with Carter's wife Hannah recommending comfort care, but she countered, "I believe in the power of prayer."

Prayer 261 (January 3, 2022)
Lord, keep us humble in your sight and in all our dealings with each other and lift us up in your due time.
We cast our anxieties on you, because you care for us.
Keep us alert – protect us from your ravenous enemy.
Give us the strength to resist him, standing firm in the faith, for your family is hunted by him throughout the world, but you are our keeper.
God of all grace, who called us to your eternal glory through Christ, restore us and make us strong and steadfast.
All power and glory are yours forever and ever.
[From 1 Peter 6-10]

I was in an ICU room with a Covid patient that needed intubation and a physician I had never seen before came in and started giving orders. I had no idea what they were doing in here – this was *my* ICU, *my patient*. I told them I had things under control and didn't need their help. They silently stood aside, but I could feel their cool gaze on the back of my neck as I rushed ahead – their presence for some reason prompting me into precipitous action. The ETT was inserted down the patient's throat in a moment. I straightened up to look at my work.

Something was wrong.

The patient wasn't connected to a ventilator. Somehow, I had intubated without any equipment, without any nurses or RTs – the patient wasn't even receiving oxygen!

For a moment though, everything seemed OK – the patient breathing on their own through the ETT. Suddenly, they sat up in bed and looked me right in the eye, terror dawning. It seemed like they were trying to say something of the utmost importance to me, but the ETT had rendered them mute. Suddenly, the ETT filled with a solid column of bright red arterial blood that spewed out all over the bed! The patient couldn't draw a single further breath, couldn't even scream. They slumped forward and the blood poured out of the tube over the side of the bed, pulsing bright, then darkening as the puddle quickly expanded across the linoleum floor.

I woke momentarily disoriented. Hot and sweaty, I pulled the sheets off and quietly lay in bed awhile, cooling off and letting my pulse settle. I waited awhile longer . . . longer, but sleep wouldn't come. I started thinking about my patient list, prioritizing the tasks of my next work shift starting in just a few hours; then I relived Cliff's code arrest, got angry again over what had been done to Salvatore. *I wished I could just turn my darn brain off!*

I turned on my Kindle and started reading *Cold Mountain* by Charles Frazier until I couldn't keep my eyelids open. I dropped the Kindle, closed my eyes, and silently recited Psalm 23 over and over until I fell back asleep.

Prayer 262 (January 4, 2022)
You have done a new thing.
It has sprung up, though we are slow to see.
You have made a way in the desert, a stream in the wasteland.
Yet only a few have called out to you.
We have made no sacrifice to you, though we have burdened you
with our sins and wearied you with our offenses.

You command us to state the case for our innocence.
You have given us the answer: "The Cross!"
Now Jesus himself blots out our transgressions, for your sake, and
remembers our sins no more.
Praise be to God!
[Modern interpretation of Isaiah 43, part 2]

I met Carter's wife Hannah on a nightshift I covered for Joyce, who had called-in sick with a mild case of Covid. An administrative milestone had passed since the last time I worked: family visitation had been restored for Covid patients sick for more than three weeks, at which point they were highly likely to no longer be contagious. When I arrived at work, the nurses warned me that Hannah and their daughter Tess had been waiting in Carter's room for the doctor to arrive – Hannah had some new suggestions for Carter's medical care that she wanted to discuss. *Just what I needed!*

I looked over Carter's chart carefully before heading over to meet her so that I could be prepared. Carter had been slowly deteriorating in the ICU since his admission 29 days earlier. He was on 90% oxygen and requiring heavy sedation. But I noted a few therapeutic opportunities: Carter's weight was up 12 kg since admission, suggesting that he might be fluid-overloaded. A build-up of fluid in his lungs was a problem that could be solved by giving a diuretic to increase his urine output. Carter had completed a 10-day course of standard dexamethasone therapy over two weeks ago – we could try another, *higher* dose course of steroids.

Carter's room had been decorated by his family like some families used to do in the days before Covid. I had forgotten how nice that was. Pictures were taped in a row along the wall facing his bed: four generations of his family dressed in jeans, T-shirts and cowboy hats, assorted farm animals (mostly horses and cows – *my favorite a very cute black calf*) and about a dozen hand-written gospel verses. A dusty well-worn black ten-gallon cowboy hat was on the bedside table. I introduced myself to Hannah and Tess, "It's really nice what you ladies did to Carter's room, lets us know who he really is and who loves him – you even brought his cowboy hat in!"

"That would be my hat!" Tess answered matter-of-factly. She had on the stiffest, darkest-blue pair of Levi's jeans seen since stone-washing was invented. I didn't even know they still sold them that way anymore. Her smile lit up the room. Hannah handed me a phone number to call – a doctor she knew who had made the (preposterous) contention that Carter would recover if only we treated him with 3% saline (salt water) intravenously. I didn't even try to argue. I could sense right away that things were different now – we could communicate in a fundamentally better way in person than we ever could over the phone.

"Hannah – I appreciate this phone number (folding and putting it in my pocket), but I think I can say without bragging that I have more than my share of experience with Covid, and I keep up to date with the legitimate research. I can tell you without any doubt that 3% saline won't help Carter. But I have been looking through his chart, and there *are* a few new things that I want to try for him. I explained my plans to try diuretics and another, higher–dose course of steroids. Finally I said, "I hope you and Tess can trust me with Carter's care, and believe me when I tell you, I will treat Carter as though he was my brother."

Hannah smiled. "Ah, but Dr. Eckshar, he *is* your brother."

Smiles all around. Restoration of visitation would quickly heal our rapport with many of our families over the next few weeks. For me, that process started on this visit. Hannah, Tess and I prayed out loud in Carter's room for Lord to heal Carter, bless his family, and smile on the new treatments we were going to try. We traded cell phone numbers and Hannah started texting me gospel messages each day.

The first one was Luke 5:5: Simon answered, "Master, we've worked hard all night and haven't caught anything. But because you say so, I will let down the nets."

I texted back: "Hannah, you sharing this scripture today is no coincidence. The Lord put it on our hearts to try again in his name. More important than any new medicine, we came *together* to him on our knees. I have to believe God is now guiding our steps forward."

Prayer 263 (January 9, 2022)
Lord, our human bodies are weak, but our souls are filled with your all-surpassing spirit.
We are hard-pressed on every side but not crushed, perplexed but not in despair, persecuted but not abandoned, struck down but not destroyed.
This all-surpassing power is not from us, but from God, who said, "Let light shine out of darkness" to reveal the knowledge of God's glory reflected in the face of our Lord Jesus Christ.
Our human bodies carry death, for you did not even spare your own Son from this, but we follow in your steps Lord Jesus.
Just as you suffered and died to be born again, we are given over to death for your purpose, so that you can pour abundant life into our mortal bodies.
Therefore, we do not lose heart.
For our momentary afflictions are building blocks of God's eternal glory, that we will one day share.
So we fix our eyes not on what is seen, but on what is unseen.
Because what we see is temporary, but what is unseen is eternal.
[Another interpretation of 2 Corinthians 4:7-18]

Carter made slow but steady improvement each of the four days since Hannah, Tess and I first prayed together at his bedside. His urine output was copious and his oxygen requirement fell to 50%. We started withdrawing sedation to allow him to begin breathing on his own again. In an administrative miracle – *perhaps the rarest kind* – Sophie had finagled medical insurance for Carter! His hospital expenses would otherwise have been catastrophic to the finances of their family-owned ranch.

When I rounded on Carter this morning, Hannah was in the

room watching over things. Isaiah was excited because Carter seemed to be waking up as sedation was withdrawn. Hannah looked on as I examined Carter. His eyelids flickered at my voice. He wouldn't squeeze my hands when I asked him to, but he grimaced and withdrew his right arm when I pinched his right index fingernail. He similarly withdrew his right leg and his left leg, but when I pinched the fingernails of his left hand, he didn't grimace or withdraw it. I pinched harder – nothing. Hannah was looking on with growing concern. *It didn't take a doctor to know this wasn't a good sign.* After all I had seen, I didn't think this could be anything other than a stroke. How my heart sunk, all Carter's progress would be blighted if he was left severely disabled. How would he ever be able to run his ranch with a paralyzed arm?

I told Hannah we would check a CT scan emergently and get neurology on board. We each took one of Carter's hands. Isaiah joined us. I started and Hannah finished our prayer:

God – we have been putting our trust in you every day here in the ICU. We're not going to stop now.
There can be no disappointment, no setback, no complication that can stand in the way of your good plan for Carter.
Turn back everything in your way Lord.
Say the word and Carter will recover fully, and get home to his family.
Your word will be done. Restore him.
We wait for you Lord to do your will, in your time.
But please act now!

Hannah's prayer (as best as I can remember it):
We praise you, we thank you, loving Father, Jesus our savior.
We are certain in our faith. We <u>know</u> you will heal Carter.
I need him, the kids need him, the grandkids need him –
I'm claiming this victory for your glory right now,
with 100% confidence.
You love Carter and your word is law in Heaven and on Earth.
If it is your will – she paused* *– get him out of this hospital bed and*

back home to the ranch with us.
We pray in the holy name of Jesus, our savior and our healer.
[*I thought Hannah might balk here and pray for the strength to accept God's will in case Carter didn't recover, but I was wrong again. Hannah never prayed for anything less than every good thing she wanted, and that she knew God would deliver.]

Prayer 264 (January 12, 2022)
Lord, I was wandering in the wilderness, lost and alone.
But you were not willing that I should perish.
You left the 99 and came into the hills searching for me.
You found me out and rejoiced in me.
You lifted me up high on your shoulders, carried me above the thorns and sharp stones, back to your fold.
You brought me sure-footed along hidden paths only you know, to the place where I belong, the place you created me to abide in – your home.
[Adaptation of Matthew 18:12-14]

Contrary to what I believed to be a foregone conclusion, Carter's CT scan and subsequent MRI scan showed no stroke. This was of course a great relief but also a source of bewilderment. The paralysis of Carter's arm was unexplained. Neurology surmised it might be a peripheral nerve injury, but there was no history of arm trauma, and an MRI of Carter's nerve plexus appeared normal. Neurology didn't know how to explain this.

I had to wonder once again what miracles have been overlooked because we don't think they are possible. Could it be that Carter *had* a stroke and had been restored in answer to prayer? I shared this idea with Hannah and Tess, and of course that made three votes for a miracle.

Carter became increasingly interactive over the next few days. He could barely move his left arm at first, but made steady progress with the occupational therapists and eventually fully regained sensation and strength in his arm.

Prayer 265 (January 14, 2022)
God, you are love, and all love comes from you.
And this is how you showed us what love is: you sent your one and only Son into the world to save us.
We can't see you Lord, but abide in our hearts, make your love complete in us and it will shine out from us for all to see.
This is how your love is proven: that you gave us confidence for the day of judgment.
In this world, you have made us to be like Jesus, and your love for us drives out fear.
There is no fear in your love.
Our faith is the victory that has overcome the world.
Who is the one that overcomes death?
Only the one who believes that Jesus is the Son of God.
[From 1 John 4,5]

Prayer 266 (January 20, 2022)
Lord Jesus, bless your people.
We have been comforted in our distress and affliction by your gift of faith, and we survived all adversity, standing shoulder to shoulder, fast in the Lord.
How can we thank you enough for the joy we share being together with you?
We pray night and day that you will keep us strong in our faith until we see you face to face.
Lord, direct our way to you and make us abound in love for each other so that you can establish our hearts as blameless and holy before our God and Father when we stand before him at your side.
[Based on 1 Thessalonians 3:7-13]

We had admitted PJ and Carter on the same date and they recovered in parallel. Now, 47 days later, we performed tracheostomies for both of them on the same day. Within a few more days they were each discharged to rehabilitation facilities, apparently on the road to recovery.

Seven of the 28 patients in our ICU on January 15, 2021, had

Covid pneumonia. Over the next week, six died and one was transferred out to a long-term acute care facility, having barely survived despite suffering a major stroke. As these seven ICU beds were vacated, a quiet miracle occurred: they were not immediately re-occupied by other Covid patients. It took a few more weeks before we dared say it out loud, but it looked like the Delta/Omicron Covid surge was finally over.

Prayer 267 (January 27, 2022)
What if God, desiring to make known the fury of his wrath, patiently endured a people born of wrath, prepared for destruction, in order to contrast the riches of his glory bestowed on children of his mercy, whom he created to share in his kingdom?
Thank you, Lord, for creating us to be children of your mercy; sending us your Son to shoulder your wrath on our account, so that we could be made clean.
Jesus became one of us to fulfill your plan that we should be pleasing in your eyes.
Glory to you and praise and thanks for the life of Christ
[taken from Romans 9:14-26]

Things around the ICU were "returning to normal" *if there is such a thing in the ICU.*

I admitted Bella, a 39-year-old lady with end-stage coronary heart disease and heart failure (accumulation of fluid in her lungs). She didn't take her heart medications and was an avid cigarette smoker. To my amazement, she freely admitted that she regularly smoked methamphetamine – the worse possible thing she could do to her crippled heart. When I met Bella, I was forthright about the critical situation she was in, explained what we could do to help her and what *she* needed to do if she wanted to live to see 40.

Bella started crying; I first thought because of the dire situation. But when I asked what was wrong, she said her IV hurt. I examined the IV in her forearm closely: it looked fine. It wasn't infected and nothing was infusing through it (some IV medications cause pain during infusion). Bella tearfully asked for "something strong" for the pain, an awkward request as I couldn't countenance giving her strong painkillers for something as simple as an IV. Our subsequent debate demolished any rapport I might have built.

When I checked in with Bella about a half hour later, she didn't mention the IV, and I got around to asking her preferences regarding end-of-life measures, a necessary question given her near-terminal condition. Bella said, "Do everything you can to keep me alive as long as possible."

Prayer 268 (February 2, 2022)
Jesus – true light – who brought light to the world; we praise you!
You were in the world; you made the world, yet the world did not know you.
You came to your own, and your own people did not receive you.
But to all who did receive you, who believed in your name, you gave the right to become children of God, born not of blood, nor the will of the man, but of God!
[From John 1:9-14]

My acquaintance with Bella was still fresh in my memory when I met Ava, a woman in her early 50s with metastatic uterine cancer, admitted for debulking surgery of the cancer metastases painfully compressing her spinal cord. Ava had been compliant throughout twelve years of surgery, chemotherapy and radiation therapy. When I entered her room to introduce myself, I interrupted a FaceTime phone call she was having with her four-year-old granddaughter. I felt terrible about that, but Ava said she would call her granddaughter Olivia right back as soon as we were done. After I examined her, I asked about her grandkids. She patted the bed next to her. "Sit!" she made me take a load off my feet and listen awhile. She had nine grandchildren! Her most cherished victory against cancer was that she had got to see them growing up.

I got to know Ava a little better over the next three days, as she experienced a series of unfortunate post-op complications, including a blood clot in her leg and a bleeding stomach ulcer. No matter what, she smiled at each person to enter her room, downplaying these setbacks and what I had to assume was her considerable pain. Each day when I asked how she was doing, she made fists, took on a boxing stance and assumed feigned truculence. I held my palms out and she landed some pretty good little punches into them.

When I asked her about code status she replied, "Despite all this junk," wagging the IV lines hanging out of both her forearms, "I don't want to be on machines. I had a good life. When it looks like my time is near, I'm going home on hospice, so I can be with my family. Not that I don't like you and the nurses Dr. Eckshar, but I'd rather be home!" she smiled.

I had a notion about her, "Ava, let me ask you something – you are such a brave and wonderful person to be around, even after all you've been through, and what you are facing – what is your secret?"

Her ever-present smile got even bigger as she replied, "I just try to enjoy every day God gives me, in whatever way I can. It might be reading a good book, enjoying my coffee, looking out at the beautiful sky," pointing out the window of her ICU room (a view of the flat roof of an adjacent ancillary building, crisscrossed with air-conditioner ducts, but with an unbroken cerulean sky above). "Even the joy of talking with a nice person like yourself. I just try to be thankful to God each day for whatever *good things* come my way."

There is a saying in the ICU: "Only the nicest people get cancer." I think perhaps, being inescapably confronted with impending mortality, some people spiritually overcome terminal diseases by choosing to accept and appreciate happiness in whatever form each day provides - perhaps the truest manifestation of wisdom.

Whatever is true, whatever is honorable, whatever is right, whatever is pure, whatever is lovely, whatever is of good repute, if there is any excellence and if anything worthy of praise, dwell on these things. [Philippians 4:8]

It reminded me again of Dom - *I still thought of him almost daily*. Ava's spirit of wisdom was akin to that which had restored Dom's happiness. Before his passing, Dom overcame his burnout by concentrating on faith, family (his daughters and granddaughter) and his personal motto: "Carpe diem." He became satisfied with himself and his situation; although neither was perfect, he had much to be grateful for. I realized I still had a few things to learn from Dom. I pulled out my phone and scrolled down to a text from May 12, 2017 - *the last message I ever received from Dom*: "Focus on becoming happy. You've achieved much. Become satisfied with where you are. - Novak, Zen Master. (P.S. Mountain bike in shop, otherwise would ride with you this weekend.)"

My old friend and mentor, enjoying life with his granddaughter Elle.

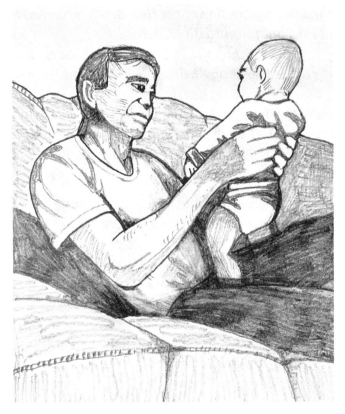

Prayer 269 (February 7, 2022)

Lord Jesus, I rejoice because I know that through prayer, your sacrifice and God's provision of the Holy Spirit, what has happened to me will turn out for my deliverance.

I eagerly expect and hope that I will be unashamed, and have sufficient courage so that Christ will be exalted in my life, and when the day comes, by my death.

For if I die with you, I know I will also be raised with you and be at your side under the Father's roof forever.

[Interpretation of Philippians 1:9-26, for someone like me – afraid to die.]

Jean and I were watching one of our favorite TV shows after dinner. I keep waiting (so far in vain) for Yellowstone's John Dutton to say a heartfelt prayer instead of taking a shot of bourbon when troubles arise. But prayer is conspicuously absent in our news or entertainment media.

However, I've come to think prayer quietly pervades our society to a much greater extent than our media depicts. Over the past years, I have asked hundreds of families to pray together in the ICU. They commonly replied they were *already* praying and had many friends and family praying as well. Almost everyone gratefully accepted prayer when offered, nurses and RTs included. Some are likely foxhole Christians, but I don't think Jesus minds *why* we come to him; in fact, he seems to love his prodigal daughters and sons the best. We shouldn't be ashamed of our faith, especially in times of distress. We are stronger when we are open about it and share it. God listens when our prayers are joined; "for where two or three are gathered together in my name, there am I in the midst of them." (Matthew 18:19-20.)

Prayer 270 (February 13, 2022)

Father Yahweh, you sacrificed your Son for us – the unworthy, the self-centered, the rebellious!

Lord Jesus, you suffered humiliation, torture and death nailed to a

cross, to reconcile us with your heavenly Father.
Now, by your grace, we the undeserving have been chosen to have a
clean heart, washed by your blood.
We will not give up what you have done for us!
We believe in you Jesus! We praise you Father God!
We dedicate this day to your service.
Just give us some work and the Holy Spirit to guide us.

There are certain unspoken rules to being a doctor, perhaps never explicitly taught, but which we all nevertheless know and rarely violate. We are not supposed to get too close to our patients, never to share our personal cell phone number, never to say sorry – *a lawyer might interpret the latter as an admission of malpractice.* Of course, praying together is so far out in left field that a specific rule prohibiting it isn't necessary.

One such rule is not to express any emotion in our documentation – just the facts. I had pretty much thrown all these rules out the window a long time ago but was surprised to learn how important violating the least could be to a patient.

This happened when we admitted a patient named Charlotte for sepsis due to a urinary tract infection. I recognized Charlotte right away – had taken care of her at the beginning of the Delta surge the previous fall. She survived a 30-day ICU admission for Covid pneumonia, during which she was sedated and barely conscious. Thankfully, most patients have little or no memory of events that occur under such circumstances and I couldn't imagine that she would have any idea we had met before. But when I walked into her room and introduced myself, her face lit up with a smile when she saw my nametag, like we were long-lost buddies. "Dr. Eckshar, I'm *so* glad to see you!"

Turns out, Charlotte didn't remember my face, and she remembered my name only because it appeared in her chart. After surviving her brush with Covid pneumonia, She was discharged to a long-term acute care facility (LTAC), trached and PEGed. She was so weak she was quadriplegic for all practical purposes and had little or no memory of how she got that way. She survived two codes at the LTAC. As she slowly recovered over months, she requested and studied her hospital records, trying to come to terms with what had happened to her. The reason she remembered my name was because of the last note I had written in her chart near the end of her ICU admission.

Charlotte recalled: "It was really hard getting back on my feet. Even after I got home, I was so weak, still on oxygen. I could barely walk. I had bed sores on my heels, fell and broke some ribs. After that, every breath I took hurt. My husband Jim had PTSD because of all that happened to us. Sometimes he would cry out my name in the middle of the night, having a nightmare that I was still dying in the hospital. I got ahold of my records. I read all your notes. And in your last note you wrote, ' Charlotte nods her head yes and no!' *With an exclamation point at the end!*"

"You see? It meant something to you! That exclamation point showed me that you cared. You wrote you were sorry someone else was going to do my tracheostomy because you wanted to do it yourself. You said it was clear that I had a 'good chance of surviving'. As I lay in bed reading those records, I started crying. I knew someone in that hospital cared about me, even though you were a stranger – someone I didn't remember ever meeting. I've prayed I would meet you someday, so I could tell you: Jim and I prayed the mass for you and the nurses. Our friends and family all over the country prayed for you all. God bless you."

I was choked up by then – lucky no one else was in the room. I never remember having done such a minuscule thing that meant so much to another person before. The ICU is a location of incredible emotional leverage. The smallest kindness might be remembered by a patient or family for the rest of their lives. Charlotte recovered after a short course of antibiotics and returned home to her husband Jim.

Prayer 271 (February 16, 2022)

Lord, grant me the wisdom of your Holy Spirit, a wisdom hidden from the world, but intended for your children since before time began. A wisdom that no eye has seen, no ear has heard, and no human mind can conceive, revealing the wonders you prepared for those who love you and a promise sealed by your Holy Spirit indwelling our hearts.

That Spirit now within us, (the mind of Jesus) searches all things, even the deep things of God! That Spirit never stops groaning on our behalf, interceding with you to save us.

When you search my heart Lord, find your Holy Spirit.

[Written after reading 1 Corinthians 2 and Romans 8:26]

As I was entering the hospital to work a night shift, I ran into Marg on her way out the door.

"Doctor! – *I never could get her to call me 'Anthony'* – I was hoping I would get to see you one more time before I left. I'm retiring today! This was my last shift!"

It took a moment for that to sink in. "Marg – I'm so happy we bumped into each other so I could say goodbye! I'm sure going to miss you. Can I give you a hug?" She smiled and we embraced a bit awkwardly (human resources policies notwithstanding).

"Now who's going to bring me pizza and ice cream?"

"Oh Doctor!" (I actually think she blushed.)

"Hey, did you ever get your vaccine?"

"Oh, yes Doctor!"

"Good. Marg, you have been such a blessing to us all – thanks so much for all your hard work and for being such a kind person. Now you deserve to put your feet up and relax! You earned it." I smiled.

"Thank you Doctor – you take care now." Marg headed out the door for home and I headed into the hospital, wondering how many of the walking-wounded on our team would leave the unit now that the Covid ICU nightmare was over. No doubt, many of us were hanging on by our fingernails, trying not to let their teammates down – but the *obligation* to stay was fading.

I wondered about Mayfield who seemed like he *almost* burned out, Joyce who endured incredible hardship but kept things to herself, Carlos – *73 years old now* – Samantha, Lynn, Isaiah and the other nurses, Sophie and Javier and June, and all the others who had suffered alongside our Covid ICU patients and their families for two long years. How many would follow Marg out the hospital door?

I even wondered about myself. Could I keep going? Was there still a human being in here somewhere if you took away the scrubs and stethoscope? I hadn't had the opportunity to seriously consider this before.

Nor did I have time for any more wool-gathering right now. I had to get to work. I supposed only time would tell.

Prayer 272 (February 18, 2022)
This is the day Carter went home to his ranch, and he and his wife Hannah sent our ICU team this prayer:

I thank God for you and I pray for you.
I have witnessed before God your work, produced by faith, your labor prompted by love, and your endurance inspired by hope in our Lord Jesus Christ.
I know you are loved by God, that he has chosen you, because our gospel came to you not simply with words but also with power, with the Holy Spirit and deep conviction.
You welcomed Christ's message in the midst of severe suffering with the joy given by the Holy Spirit, and so you became a model to all the rest of us believers.
The Lord's message rang out from you.
And your life shows how you turned from false idols to serve the living and true God, and to wait for his Son from Heaven, whom he raised from the dead —Jesus, who has rescued you and all believers from death. [1 Thessalonians 1:4-10]

Late that evening, I laid down in bed feeling more relaxed than I had in I-can't-remember-when. My mind wandered. I thought about how the sum of everything that happens to us in life – every choice we make, every belief we hold true – is what makes us who we are. These comprise our soul with a dynamic complexity far greater than that could ever be determined by our DNA. We shape each others' souls by the way we share in each other's lives.

I brought to mind all the people who carried me over the past two years: Jean, my partners, the nurses, the patients and their families. The times we shared had gravely wounded us, yet strengthened our sense of togetherness and our faith. Now, it seemed like something tremendous was all coming to an end. I felt an overwhelming sense of fulfillment and peace. My skin tingled all over and flushed with a warm frisson of appreciation. Strange as it sounds, the thought crossed my mind that I could have died happily at that moment.

I abandoned my philosophical meandering and my immediate surroundings crytstalized into sharp focus. Jean was lying silently beside me in bed. I could smell her hair, make out the almost microscopically-fine lanugo hairs of her cheek backlit by the Kindle she was reading – *likely another Nora Roberts romance novel*. The jugular venous pulsations in her neck rose and fell with the rhythm of her lifeblood.

I had *The Long Walk* by Richard Bachman on my bedside table. We would read awhile. When we got tired enough, we would pray together and fall asleep side by side. I closed my eyes, *just for a moment. The Lord is my shepherd; I shall not want...* The soft cotton sheets rustled against my skin, stirred by the gentle currents of the cast-iron ceiling fan – its quiet, reassuring rumble interrupted only by the intermittent chirping of a single cricket out in the yard – the last things I remembered before I fell into a dreamless sleep.

May 2022. *Carter back in the saddle.*

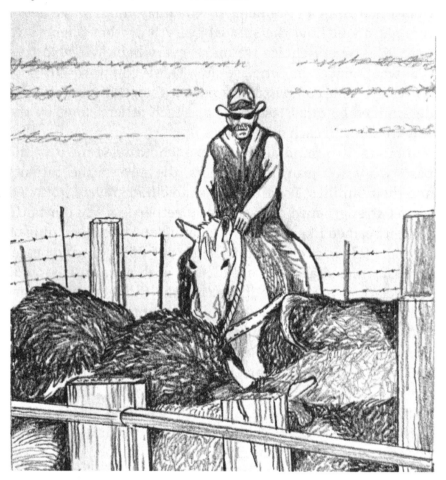

EPILOGUE

Although Covid continued to circulate in the community, it lost much of its lethality by the end of February 2022. Maybe the Delta and Omicron surges naturally immunized those who refused voluntary vaccination. Maybe the virus evolved according to God's design. Whatever the explanation, we rarely saw more than a patient or two with Covid in the ICU thereafter.

* * *

In a little less than two years, my partners and I had seen 882 critically ill Covid pneumonia patients requiring life support, cumulatively accounting for 5,839 ICU days and 4,608 ventilator days. Four hundred and two (45%) of our Covid pneumonia patients died – five times our pre-pandemic ICU mortality rate. But as high as this calculated mortality rate sounds, no one in our ICU readily accepted the figure. Mortality seemed almost universal in our collective memory, and it was only with effort we could recall our few successes. Perhaps this was because many Covid survivors passed through the ICU briefly, whereas those who died typically did so only after weeks of suffering and disappointment – burned into our memories.

None of us were particularly surprised when a research study reported that Arizona had sustained the highest adjusted Covid mortality rate in the United States – comparable with the hardest-hit countries in the world, Peru and Bulgaria.

Heatmap of adjusted Covid mortality rates in the 50 States. Adjustment is made for age, and comorbidities. [From Bollyky TJ, Castro E, Aravkin AY, et al. Assessing COVID-19 pandemic policies and behaviours and their economic and educational trade-offs across US states from Jan 1, 2020, to July 31, 2022: an observational analysis. Lancet 2023;401:1341-1360. DOI:https://doi.org/10.1016/S0140-6736(23)00461-0 Used under Creative Commons user license (Creativecommons.org)]

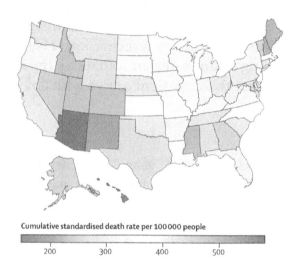

Cumulative standardised death rate per 100 000 people

200   300   400   500

There is no doubt that my time in the Covid ICU was the most difficult experience of my life. I'm not the kind of person who typically questions *why* God lets such things happen, but the question demands some explanation. The stories recounted above provide some personal answers. Covid forced me to choose. I decided to believe – the most important choice of my life. I needed adversity to quit being lukewarm, to come down on the side of faith and cry out to God, *the very thing he created me to do.* I prayed because of Covid, and God answered. By the end, I no longer had any doubt of that. I had seen too many miracles to leave any room for doubt.

I came to understand the meaning of the scripture: *"In all things God works for the good of those who love him, who have been called according to his purpose."* [Romans 8:28-30]. Covid gave me purpose – a place in God's plan, serving my sisters and brothers. Covid made me love my patients whatever their prior mistakes – *no worse than my own.* Covid taught me that faith isn't something I will ever fully possess, but rather a gift that God provides in the measure needed each moment we pray to him for it.

Ultimately, God likely has much more profound reasons than the ones I personally experienced for allowing Covid to happen – *how can there be light without darkness?* – but these were enough for me.

For those few of you still reading this book – thank you for letting me share these stories with you. Getting them off my chest certainly was part of my healing. I hope my prayers bring glory to God and encourage your faith.

One final historical acknowledgment: to steadfast King David for writing the Psalms – *placed in your heart by the Lord* – a source of solace to us all in our darkest days. I doubt you could have written them if God hadn't allowed bad things to happen to you for a brief time here on Earth.

"May his name endure forever; may it continue as long as the sun. Then all nations will be blessed through him, and they will call him blessed.
Praise be to the Lord God, the God of Israel, who alone does marvelous deeds.
Praise be to his glorious name forever; may the whole Earth be filled with his glory. Amen and Amen."
This concludes the prayers of David, son of Jesse. [Psalm 72]

MEDICAL GLOSSARY

Glossary of medical terms and abbreviations used in this book.

Advanced cardiac life support (ACLS) is a standardized protocol used to resuscitate a patient experiencing a cardiopulmonary arrest (or a "code"). ACLS includes chest compressions, oxygen administration, ventilatory (breathing) support, life support medications, heart monitoring and electrical heart shocks in some cases. Some minor surgical procedures are included when necessary, such as the placement of a chest tube in a patient with a ruptured lung. Bedside doctors and nurses refer to providing ACLS as "coding the patient."

Ambu bag is the commonly-used proprietary name for a device for manually providing breathing support to a patient. It consists of an oval mask that seals around the patient's nose and mouth, attached to a squeezable 1-liter air bag constantly filled by an oxygen source. When the mask is firmly held over the patient's face and the bag is squeezed, a breath of oxygen is pushed into the patient's lungs through their nose and mouth. An Ambu bag is used temporarily to breathe for a patient until a more long-term method such as intubation and mechanical ventilation is initiated (see below).

Bi-level Positive Airway Pressure (BiPAP) is a form of breathing life support. BiPAP is delivered by a very tight-fitting mask that covers the patient's nose and mouth, attached to a ventilator that provides a modest level of back pressure while the patient exhales, and a higher pressure to help them inhale. BiPAP can also be beneficial in non–ICU applications, such as in patients with sleep apnea who use it at home at night.

Borborygmi are bowel sounds including farts. This term wasn't used in the book – I just included it to give whoever put the effort into reading this glossary something funny to tell their kids or grandkids.

Cardiopulmonary arrest (or colloquially: "code") is the term used to describe when a patient stops breathing or loses their pulse as a potential prelude to death, which may yet be averted if ACLS is quickly started and successful. "Calling the code" refers to stopping ACLS when the code team determines that ongoing resuscitation is futile; this usually occurs if a pulse is not restored after approximately 20 minutes of ACLS.

A **Chest tube** is a long plastic tube placed into the space between the chest wall and lung and attached to a suction device to drain out abnormal fluid or air caused by a variety of diseases. We saw many patients with severe Covid pneumonia whose lungs ruptured under the pressure of mechanical ventilation – the medical term for this is "pneumothorax" – *ancient Greek for "air-chest."* Air from the ruptured lung is trapped inside the chest and prevents the lung from inflating, causing it to collapse. A chest tube can remove the air and allow the damaged lung to re-expand.

Comfort care is a treatment regimen focused on providing relief of symptoms rather than on prolonging life at all costs (*referring to the cost of human suffering*). Comfort care is appropriately administered to patients who have little to no chance of achieving outcomes they would personally find acceptable as a result of aggressive medical care. Patients receiving comfort care also have a DNR status (see below) and have invasive life support such as mechanical ventilation discontinued. Life support would never be withdrawn without also providing comfort care unless the patient is already deceased.

Cardiopulmonary resuscitation (CPR) is the most essential component of ACLS, consisting of chest compressions to pump blood to the brain and other organs, *plus* breathing support, typically given via an Ambu bag in the hospital setting. The aim of CPR is to keep the patient alive until the other elements of ACLS have a chance to enable the return of a natural pulse.

Do-not-resuscitate (DNR) is an order, generally based on the preference of the patient (expressed directly or via an appropriate surrogate) that directs medical staff to allow natural death in the event of cardiopulmonary arrest. A patient with a DNR order will not receive CPR, ACLS, cardiac shock or intubation. A wide spectrum of appropriate medical care can still be provided to a patient with a DNR order, and many DNR patients respond favorably to hospital care and survive until discharge to live another day.

Delirium tremens (DTs) is the severest form of alcohol withdrawal, usually beginning about 72 hours after abstinence and characterized by tremors, delusions, hallucinations, hypertension, tachycardia (fast heart rate), physical agitation, and in some cases, seizures. DTs are difficult to prevent and treat, sometimes requiring humongous doses of sedation drugs such as valium. The care of a patient with DTs is extremely time-consuming and challenging for their nurse.

An **Echocardiogram** is an ultrasound of the heart. These can be done at bedside by an ICU doctor in order to obtain information on how the various chambers and valves of the heart are working. This information is particularly useful in patients in shock.

Extracorporeal membrane oxygenation (ECMO) is the highest conventional form of life support. The ECMO machine pulls approximately 4-5 liters of blood (practically the entire volume of blood in the human body) per minute through a membrane that adds oxygen into the blood. The oxygenated blood can be returned upstream from the lungs, taking over their essential function, or downstream from the heart – *essentially taking the place of the lungs and heart!* ECMO is only provided at select hospitals with special expertise in its application.

The **Electronic medical record (EMR)** contains information regarding the patient's identity, demographics, past medical history, medications, physician and nursing notes, laboratory and radiography results. Access to the EMR is highly protected by security technology in accordance with federal HIPAA (Health Information Portability and Accountability Act) regulations. The colloquialism "charting" used in this book refers to accessing data from the EMR and writing notes and orders on it.

Emergency medical service (EMS), also known as paramedic service, is a team of mobile frontline healthcare providers who commonly provide initial treatment and/or resuscitation to severely ill patients who can't make it to the hospital on their own, stabilizing them and safely transporting them to the hospital.

An **Endotracheal tube (ETT)** is a clear plastic tube about as thick around as your finger and 30cm long. ETTs are placed down the patient's throat and into their lungs to connect them to a mechanical ventilator in a procedure called intubation (see below).

Extubation (or colloquially: "pulling the tube") is the procedure in which an endotracheal tube (ETT) is removed, allowing the patient to breathe on their own. Great care is taken in the timing of extubation. Leaving the ETT in too long can lead to secondary bacterial pneumonia. Removing it before the patient is ready to breathe on their own can potentially be fatal if difficulties arise replacing the ETT.

Fiberoptic bronchoscopy is the passage of a lighted, flexible fiberoptic instrument down the windpipe and into the lungs to suction deep secretions, unblock the internal airways and collect specimens for microbiological studies.

A **High-flow nasal cannula** is a special type of oxygen delivery device that fits in the patient's nostrils and can deliver 100% oxygen. A high-flow nasal cannula incorporates a device that rapidly humidifies the oxygen, allowing up to 60 liters per minute to be delivered without drying out the patient's throat. This was a Godsend for patients with severe Covid pneumonia who didn't quite require intubation, as it allows the patient to eat, drink and converse, unlike the more intrusive BiPAP mask.

Intubation (also: endotracheal intubation, or colloquially: "tubing the patient") is the procedure in which an endotracheal tube is passed through the patient's mouth and vocal cords into the windpipe of the lungs (the trachea). The patient is heavily sedated for this procedure. Problems occurring during intubation are imminently life-threatening, and it is a procedure all ICU doctors perform with trepidation.

Mechanical ventilation is a form of life support in which a machine attached to an ETT either assists or completely takes over the breathing of a critically ill patient. A ventilator uses pressure to inflate the lungs during inspiration. In general, the sicker the patient's lungs become, the more pressure is required. In patients with severe pneumonia ventilator pressures have to be limited to avoid causing further damage to the lungs.

An **N95 facemask** is a facemask that filters out 95% of particles the size of airborne pathogens such as Covid. N95 masks were recommended to be worn while providing care to Covid patients. They provide better filtration than simple surgical facemasks utilized for "universal masking" in the hospital, but they are less comfortable to wear over long periods.

Oxygen saturation (O2 sat) is the percentage of hemoglobin in arterial blood carrying oxygen. Hemoglobin in red blood cells is designed to carry large amounts of oxygen. The higher the percentage of hemoglobin carrying oxygen, the more oxygen is delivered to the brain, heart, and other organs of the body. O2 sats are normally >95%. With Covid pneumonia, an O2 sat <92% would indicate that a patient should be seen in an emergency room. An O2 sat <90% requires the administration of supplemental oxygen. O2 sats in the 80–90% range are generally considered unacceptable and if they persist despite oxygen supplementation, indicate the need for more aggressive respiratory support.

Oxygen delivery is required when a patient with a medical condition, for instance pneumonia, experiences a fall in their O2 sat to 90% or lower. Supplemental oxygen is delivered by nasal cannula, BiPAP or a ventilator. Patients with Covid pneumonia in the ICU generally require lots of supplemental oxygen, in the range of 40–100%, ramped up as needed to maintain O2 sat above 90%. For comparison, natural air has 21% oxygen.

A **P100 mask** is a facemask that filters out more than 99.9% of particles the size of airborne particles of pathogens such as Covid, making the P100 virtually impenetrable as long as it is properly worn. It was the best protection we had against Covid in the ICU until vaccination became available.

A **Pulmonary embolism (PE)** is a blood clot originating in one of the veins of the body, most commonly in the upper leg, that breaks free and floats through the veins, lodging in the lungs. PEs can cause sudden cardiopulmonary arrest if they block a significant proportion of the blood vessels of the lungs, overwhelming the ability of the heart to pump blood through them. Treatment of PE involves the use of blood thinners such as heparin.

Positive end–expiratory pressure (PEEP) is a type of ventilator pressure setting. PEEP applies pressure while the patient is trying to exhale. This keeps the lungs from completely collapsing during exhalation, improving the O2 sat.

A **Percutaneous endoscopic gastrostomy (PEG)** is a feeding tube placed through the wall of the stomach with the assistance of a fiberoptic scope that visualizes the placement of the PEG from *inside* the stomach. A PEG is typically placed in severely debilitated patients not expected to be able to safely swallow food in the near term. The colloquial expression "she was PEGed" means the patient underwent placement of such a feeding tube.

Personal protective equipment (PPE) is used to protect people from contagious infectious diseases. In the case of highly infectious airborne pathogens, like Covid, PPE consists of an N95 (or better) facemask, eye protection, gown and gloves.

Pressors (or vasopressors) are potent drugs given by continuous intravenous drip to increase blood pressure when it is dangerously low. An example mentioned in the book is Levophed. These drugs act by making the muscular walls of the arteries contract and/or by increasing the strength or speed of the heartbeat. The general objective of a pressor drug is to maintain a blood pressure of at least 90/60 mmHg, necessary for blood to deliver oxygen to the brain, heart and other organs.

Proning (as in "proning bed" or "proning a patient") is the act of turning a patient face-down in bed. This position often has the effect of better balancing blood flow and oxygen distribution in the lungs resulting in an improvement in O2 sat.

A **Respiratory therapist (RT)** is a healthcare worker with expertise in the practice of administering oxygen, giving respiratory treatments, and operating ventilators.

Shock is a state in which the circulatory system fails to adequately perfuse the organs with oxygen. This is usually accompanied by severe hypotension (low blood pressure) typically less than 90/60. The term septic shock is used when shock is caused by a life-threatening infection such as severe Covid pneumonia. Shock can also be caused by severe heart failure, pulmonary embolism or a ruptured lung, among other things.

A **Speaking valve** (or Passy–Muir valve) is a small one-way valve that can be attached to the outside of a tracheostomy tube allowing the patient to speak. This is possible because the valve opens when the patient inhales, but closes when they exhale, forcing air through the vocal cords.

Supining is the opposite of proning. The supine patient is lying on their back, face-up in bed. "Supining" means turning the patient into a supine position.

Tracheostomy (or colloquially: "trach") refers to both a breathing tube and the procedure in which it is placed. A tracheostomy is a plastic tube about as long and big around as a ring finger, placed through the front of the neck under the Adam's apple into the trachea (the main windpipe of the lungs). A tracheostomy is usually placed in patients who require mechanical ventilation for more than two weeks because an endotracheal tube left in place longer than that may cause damage to the trachea. The colloquial expression, "He was trached" means the patient had a tracheostomy placed.

Universal masking is based on common sense and scientific evidence that shows that wearing a surgical mask when indoors around other people provides some protection against contagious airborne diseases. The surgical mask probably provides the most benefit by keeping airborne virus particles *exhaled by the wearer* out of the air – in other words, it's probably more important for the protection of others than for the protection of the wearer. This point is lost on anti-maskers, who seemed to feel they were being brave by refusing to wear masks; in fact, they were risking exposing the people around them to Covid if they should be infected.

Acknowledgments. My Bible study brothers and many friends who helped edit this book – *you know who you are* – I thank you.

Disclaimer. The medical errors described in this book are fictional. I admit, I made some serious non-fictional medical errors during the Covid pandemic despite my best effort and intentions. I was ashamed to share them, but they played an important role in this story that I could not simply ignore. No ICU story can be complete without sharing how deeply such mistakes affect patients and the people doing their best to take care of them.

APPENDIX: CRITICAL APPRAISAL OF MEDICAL LITERATURE 101

I wanted to provide a more detailed explanation of why my partners and I considered therapies such as hydroxychloroquine or ivermectin "unproven or disproven" and refused to administer them to Covid patients. This argument is too in-depth to repeatedly explain to angry patient family members over the phone, but it might provide interested readers with the rationale for our evidence-based Covid practice. There are three foundational concepts to consider.

1) *Nearly all* potential medical therapies that undergo rigorous testing are found *not* to benefit human beings. Researchers are very persistent in looking for solutions. They have to be, because the vast majority of proposed medical interventions turn out to be unhelpful or even harmful. A recent analysis of over 60 years of research in critical care medicine found only a handful of therapies (all associated with the use of gentler methods of mechanical ventilation) were proven to improve survival in the ICU. The chances that in our desperation, we would take an antiparasitic drug off the shelf (such as hydroxychloroquine or ivermectin) and find that it effectively treats a coronavirus is an *extreme* long shot from the get-go. These drugs have been around for many decades (hydroxychloroquine since the 1940s) and were never before found clinically beneficial for any viral infection.

Conversely, all drugs have side effects. *I recall a patient who tried to treat his AIDS with vitamins and died from an inadvertent vitamin A overdose which caused his liver to shut down.* There is a strong instinct to "just try something" in a desperate situation, but putting an unproven drug into your body is *far* more likely to make things worse than better. That's part of where the expression "First do no harm" came from. Not many people nowadays would try to fix their flatscreen TV by opening up the back and going in there with a screwdriver "just to try something" – *think how much more complicated the human body is than your TV, and how much more dangerous "sticking a screwdriver into it" might be!*

2) A high proportion of "medical research" accessible to the public is of low quality. The *traditional* model for implementing research into medical practice began when the research manuscript was submitted to a "peer-reviewed" journal. Articles were only chosen for publication if the journal editors (highly accomplished academicians) *plus* two or three independent external experts in the field agreed that the study was properly performed and that the conclusions were supported by the results. This can be a very arduous process, as I can personally attest. In one case, it took me two years to correct the analysis and conclusions of a research project to the satisfaction of my peer reviewers.

But in recent years, the process of peer review has been weakened and, in some cases, eliminated. Hundreds of internationally-based "predatory" medical journals have been founded that make their money by charging scientists for publishing their research rather than through subscription fees. The review process of such journals has an inherent financial bias to accept publication, in my opinion.

Online publication of "pre-prints" provides public access to studies that are completely unverified by peer review. Several studies that indicated a survival benefit for hydroxychloroquine and ivermectin were available to the public electronically as pre-prints but were never officially published because of glaring methodological flaws. In other cases, the supporting data was unavailable upon request by journal editors. When a researcher's data "is unavailable", it essentially suggests the data never existed. [Imagine what an IRS auditor would assume if you told them your financial records were unavailable.] But whether such studies were simply poorly devised or overtly fraudulent, they had a strong impact on public opinion during the pandemic, even if they were never officially published.

3) Most lay people (*and even many doctors*) are unpracticed in the principles of clinical epidemiology and critical appraisal necessary to decipher whether a research study was well conducted and its conclusions believable.

Clinical epidemiology is the science of *how we know what we know* in medicine. It has to do with how research is designed to elucidate associations between exposures or treatments and health outcomes. Many different research designs can be used to examine the same research question, and each has inherent weaknesses that can produce misleading results. Although any research design can be done well or poorly, there is a hierarchy of study types in clinical epidemiology that can be used to rank those most likely to be trustworthy.

The lowest tier: includes statements of opinion, case reports, animal studies, and in-vitro studies. A good example is a study that showed ivermectin reduced Covid viral replication in a test tube – *at concentrations 100 times higher than achievable in a human body*. Even "promising" in-vitro studies only very rarely lead to beneficial treatments. Cancer would have been cured a long time ago if not for this unfortunate truth.

The middle tier: case-control and cohort studies in which the researcher doesn't intervene but observes associations between risk factors or treatments and health outcomes of interest. An example is a paper that reported 54 patients with "confirmed or presumed" Covid who were treated with hydroxychloroquine and doxycycline. Forty-six recovered, six deteriorated, requiring hospitalization and three died – *yes, I know it doesn't add up*. The authors concluded that hydroxychloroquine and doxycycline were associated with clinical recovery, decreased hospitalization (11%) and improved mortality (6%) by comparing their results with those reported by another researcher from another part of the country. However, we now know that an 11% hospitalization rate and 6% mortality are not particularly encouraging results, and different patient populations have a wide variation of Covid outcomes. So it's impossible to say whether this drug combination had any benefit whatsoever. This study was never published and, therefore, never successfully underwent peer review. Low and middle-tier studies are "hypothesis-generating" – meaning they pique our interest in performing high-tier clinical research, but ought not to be used to justify giving a drug to a patient.

The highest tier comprises clinical trials in which researchers randomly assign patients to treatment versus placebo control. One poorly designed but influential clinical trial involved the administration of ivermectin to 26 Covid inpatients with comparison to 16 control patients from other institutions (not randomly chosen). *Strangely, only eight of the 42 patients had Covid pneumonia, so it wasn't clear why they were admitted to the hospital.* Twenty of the patients that received ivermectin were statistically compared to 16 controls and the ivermectin patients had a more rapid reduction in viral shedding. However, six patients that received ivermectin dropped out before the analysis – one due to intolerable side effects of ivermectin, three because they required ICU admission, and one because they died! No control patient was lost to follow-up. So it appears that the four worst clinical outcomes in the study (ICU admission or death) all occurred in the patients receiving ivermectin! Yet the author focused on the lab results, concluding that "hydroxychloroquine treatment is significantly associated with viral load reduction/ disappearance in COVID-19 patients." Clinical trials should focus on clinical rather than laboratory outcomes. *Who cares if you cleared viral shedding but didn't survive?* This small study used control patients from other institutions that were not randomly chosen and therefore introduced the potential for bias (e.g., the control group might have been more prone to delayed viral clearance for any number of reasons, for instance, higher rates of diabetes, lung or coronary disease or cancer). Ultimately, this article was published by the journal for which the author himself served as an Editor! - A clear conflict of interest.

Contrast this with the RECOVERY trial, which had an immediate impact on our patient care starting in the Summer Surge of 2020. This study, published in the New England Journal of Medicine, enrolled over 6400 patients and showed that dexamethasone reduced mortality by one-third in patients with Covid pneumonia requiring mechanical ventilation, compared to randomly chosen placebo control patients. We believed the results of this study for several reasons including: a randomized control group to avoid introducing bias, enrollment of a large sample size at multiple hospitals, use of clinical rather than laboratory outcomes, and analysis of all patients enrolled in the study. This is the type of study worth trusting in terms of administering drugs to real live persons.

If this whole appendix is boring you, you are a normal human being. The myriad details that a reader would have to dig out of the research methodology and publication history to decide whether they should accept the conclusions of a research manuscript takes the ability to suppress personal bias and a lot of knowledge, time and effort. So you can see why it is seldom done, even by doctors that once received some training in how to do it. Therefore you will hear physicians making poorly-informed public statements at times, having forgotten the basic principles of clinical epidemiology upon which our conclusions should be based.

However, a careful review of all the articles on ivermectin by international experts in critical appraisal has revealed that there is (at the time of this writing) no evidence that ivermectin works in any situation for preventing or treating Covid, based on analysis of all available global data that met acceptable quality standards. [See the Cochrane Database of Systematic Reviews for specific critical appraisal of studies regarding ivermectin for Covid and many other medical treatments if interested.]

For me, ivermectin had nothing to do with politics; my patients' lives were at stake! The evidence-based practice of medicine is achieved when the results of one or more multi-center randomized controlled trial(s) determine whether or not to give a patient a drug in clinical practice. This is the standard to which our group held ourselves throughout our careers together and we didn't let our standard slip during the pandemic.

SELECTED REFERENCES

Tomlinson B, Cockram C. SARS: experience at Prince of Wales Hospital, Hong Kong. Lancet. 2003;361:1486-1487. DOI: 10.1016/S0140-6736(03)13218-7.

Butler, D. Engineered bat virus stirs debate over risky research. Nature. 2015. DOI: 10.1038/nature.2015.18787.

Zhan, Mingkun, et al. Death from Covid-19 of 23 healthcare workers in China. N Engl J Med. 2020;382: 2267-2268. DOI: 10.1056/NEJMc2005696.

Holshue ML, DeBolt C, Lindquist S, et al; Washington State 2019-nCoV Case Investigation Team. First Case of 2019 Novel Coronavirus in the United States. N Engl J Med. 2020 Mar 5;382(10):929-936. DOI: 10.1056/NEJMoa2001191.

McMichael TM, Clark S, Pogosjans S, Kay M, et al; Public Health – Seattle & King County, Evergreen Health, and CDC COVID-19 Investigation Team. COVID-19 in a Long-Term Care Facility - King County, Washington, February 27-March 9, 2020. MMWR 2020 Mar 27;69(12):339-342. DOI: 10.15585/mmwr.mm6912e1.

Horby P, Lim WS, Emberson JR et al for the RECOVERY Collaborative Group. Dexamethasone in hospitalized patients with Covid-19. N Engl J Med. 2021;384:693.

Polack FP, Thomas SJ, Kitchin N, et al. Safety and Efficacy of the BNT162b2 mRNA Covid-19 Vaccine. N Engl J Med 2020; 383:2603-2615. DOI: 10.1056/NEJMoa2034577.

Rosenblum HG, Gee J, Liu R et al. Safety of mRNA vaccines administered during the initial 6 months of the US COVID-19 vaccination programme: an observational study of reports to the Vaccine Adverse Event Reporting System and v-safe.

Lancet Infectious Diseases. 2022;22:802-812. DOI: 10.1016/S1473-3099(22)00054-8

Saag MS. Misguided use of hydroxychloroquine for COVID-19: the infusion of politics into science. JAMA. 2020;324(21):2161–2162. DOI: 10.1001/jama.2020.22389

Popp M, Stegemann M, Metzendorf MI, et al. Ivermectin for preventing and treating COVID-19. Cochrane Database of Systematic Reviews. 2021, Issue 7. Art. No.: CD015017. DOI: 10.1002/14651858.CD015017.pub2.

Guyatt GH, Sackett DL, Cook DJ. Users' guides to the medical literature. II. How to use an article about therapy or prevention. A. Are the results of the study valid? Evidence-Based Medicine Working Group. JAMA. 1993 Dec;270(21):2598-2601. DOI: 10.1001/jama.270.21.2598. PMID: 8230645.

Bollyky TJ, Castro E, Aravkin AY, Bhangdia K, et al. Assessing COVID-19 pandemic policies and behaviors and their economic and educational trade-offs across US states from Jan 1, 2020, to July 31, 2022: an observational analysis. Lancet. Open Access. Published online: March 23, 2023 DOI:https://doi.org/10.1016/S0140-6736(23)00461-0.

Made in the USA
Las Vegas, NV
11 August 2023